YOUR COMPLETE GUIDE TO

Breast Augmentation & Body Contouring

THOMAS B. MCNEMAR, M.D. • C. ANDREW SALZBERG, M.D.

STEVEN P. SEIDEL, M.D.

Addicus Books

Omaha, Nebraska

An Addicus Nonfiction Book

ISBN#   1-886039-74-07
         978-1886039-74-2

Cover design by Peri Poloni
Illustrations by Jack Kusler
Typography by Linda Dageforde

This book is not intended to serve as a substitute for a physician.
Nor is it the authors' intent to give medical advice contrary to that of an attending physician.

Library of Congress Cataloging-in-Publication Data

McNemar, Thomas, 1962-
  Your complete guide to breast augmentation and body contouring / Thomas McNemar, C. Andrew Salzberg, Steven P. Seidel.
  p. cm.
  Includes index.
  ISBN 1-886039-74-7 (alk. paper)
  1. Augmentation mammaplasty—Popular works. 2. Liposuction—Popular works. 3. Surgery, Plastic—Popular works. I. Salzberg, C. Andrew, 1957- II. Seidel, Steven P., 1962- III. Title.

RD539.8.M44 2006
618.1'90592—dc22   2006000966

Addicus Books, Inc.
P.O. Box 45327
Omaha, Nebraska 68145
www.AddicusBooks.com

Printed in the United States of America
10 9 8 7 6 5 4 3 2 1

Contents

To my wife Cindy and my children Mackenzie and Kelsey.
May you always follow your dreams.

Thomas B. McNemar, M.D.

To Anita, Jennifer, and Emily—the women
who make my life worthwhile.

C. Andrew Salzberg, M.D.

To my wife, Bethany, and to parents, Dennis and Jeanette Seidel,
who have encouraged and supported me every step of the way.

Steven P. Seidel, M.D.

Acknowledgments

A book of this type requires many different talents. I would like to thank Rod Colvin for bringing the book together. I thank my two colleagues, Dr. Salzberg and Dr. Seidel, for their insights, and I acknowledge my staff, Tamee, Bobbie, Danielle, and Erin. I would like to thank all my patients, past and future. I also thank for my family, Cindy, Mackenzie and Kelsey. I am blessed to have them.

Thomas B. McNemar, M.D.

This book has been made possible thanks to the support and efforts of many people. First, I would like to extend my thanks and gratitude to my exceptional colleagues and staff members at the New York Group for Plastic Surgery. Their dedication and tireless efforts helped keep this project on track. I am also indebted to my patients, who provide me with inspiration on a daily basis. Finally, I would like to thank Frances Sharpe for her editorial assistance in bringing this book to life.

C. Andrew Salzberg, M.D.

I would like to thank my wife, Bethany, for her devotion and support of my professional endeavors, which have often required sacrifice on her part. I would also like to thank Marcie Jacob for undying friendship and years of intellectual stimulation. I extend my thanks for Frances Sharpe for her editorial work on this book. I also thank Tracy McMinn for assisting with the patient photographs for this book.

Steven P. Seidel, M.D.

Introduction

Once reserved for the rich and famous, cosmetic surgery has become more popular than ever. These days, millions of people from all walks of life—teachers, business executives, homemakers—are improving their looks as well as their self-image with cosmetic procedures. Among women, liposuction, breast augmentation, and tummy tucks are among the most popular surgical procedures, respectively. And the number of these procedures performed each year keeps climbing.

The explosion in aesthetic surgery has led to an increase in the number and type of physicians performing these surgeries. Never has it been more important for you to be informed about your surgery and the credentials of your surgeon.

Whether you're considering enhancing what nature gave you through breast augmentation or thinking about restoring a more youthful appearance through body contouring, we encourage you to learn as much as you can about the cosmetic procedures available to you. The better informed you are, the more likely you are to achieve the results you desire.

In this book, you'll learn about each of these popular procedures, including what to expect before and after surgery. And with dozens of before-and-after photos of our patients, you'll see firsthand the kind of results that can be achieved. We hope you will find this easy-to-understand book to be a useful resource and a starting point for you as you explore your options and make choices about breast augmentation and body contouring surgery.

CHAPTER ONE

Body Contouring Surgery: An Overview

1

Body Contouring Surgery: An Overview

*W*hen you look in a full-length mirror, are you pleased with the figure you see? Or do you notice things you'd like to change? Are there clothing styles you'd like to wear, but don't because you're not comfortable with the way your body looks? Do you wish you could do something to enhance the appearance of your physique? If so, you're not alone. Millions of Americans would like to improve their shape, and more and more of them are turning to cosmetic plastic surgery as a way to get results.

Body Contouring Procedures

What is body contouring? Body contouring refers to cosmetic surgical procedures designed to address specific abnormalities or irregularities of the chest, trunk, and extremities. Among the most common body contouring procedures for women are breast augmentation, liposuction, and abdominoplasty (also known as a tummy tuck).

What Is Breast Augmentation?

Breast augmentation is a surgical procedure that increases the size and proportions of your breasts by using breast implants. Breast-implant surgery can enhance a small bustline, correct breasts that differ in size or shape, and reshape breasts that have lost their firmness. In most cases, the procedure results in a better-proportioned figure that allows you to wear more clothing styles and, ultimately, feel more confident about yourself. According to research, women who undergo breast augmentation are happy with the results. In a 1995 study that followed breast-implant patients through the year 2000, 95 percent reported satisfaction with their breast implants five years after surgery.

What Is Liposuction?

Liposuction is a surgical procedure that can safely, effectively, and permanently remove fat from the body. The procedure is best suited to removing specific, localized fat deposits that are resistant to diet and exercise. Using this procedure, a surgeon can sculpt or reshape specific areas of the body, producing a smoother, more proportional figure.

Liposuction was first introduced to the United States in the 1980s. Since then, improvements in surgical techniques and instruments have allowed surgeons to perform the procedure more safely, to achieve better results, and to shorten the recovery period. Today, surgeons can choose from several advanced surgical techniques and instruments to help you achieve the best results.

Although liposuction can produce amazing results, there are limits to what it can achieve. Recommended guidelines limit the amount of fat that can safely be removed and the amount of body sculpting that can be accomplished. Because of this, it should not be considered a substitute for weight reduction or a treatment for obesity.

What Is a Tummy Tuck?

A tummy tuck, also called abdominoplasty, is a surgical procedure that redefines the contours of your abdomen. It can give you a flatter stomach and a more defined waistline. Like liposuction, it eliminates stubborn fat that doesn't respond to diet and exercise. But a tummy tuck goes beyond what liposuction can achieve. The procedure also creates a smoother tummy surface by removing loose skin and stretch marks. And the procedure can actually tighten stretched-out muscles of the abdominal wall (or more accurately, the connective tissues called fascia that cover the muscles), instantly creating a more defined waistline.

In addition to removing lumps and bulges, a tummy tuck may also help you shed feelings of self-consciousness about the shape of your body. Following the procedure, you may feel comfortable enough to wear a bathing suit, or you may find that you can slip into jeans you haven't worn in a decade.

Is Body Contouring Surgery for You?

If you want to regain a trimmer, more youthful-looking body or want to add a few curves to your shape, you may be a candidate for body contouring surgery. Provided you're in good overall health, remarkable improvements are possible whether you're in your twenties, your seventies, or even beyond. And regardless of whether you're tall or petite, broad-shouldered or narrow, you can emerge with a more flattering form. However, surgeons look at more than just your physical attributes when deciding if you're a good candidate for a body contouring procedure. Any qualified cosmetic plastic surgeon will also assess your expectations, your motivation, your mental health, and your willingness to take an active role in the process.

Attitude and Expectations

Having realistic expectations is one of the most important qualifications for anyone seeking a cosmetic procedure. Cosmetic surgeons stress that body contouring procedures generally result in improvements rather than perfection. If you understand and accept this fact, you're far more likely to be satisfied with your results.

Following body contouring surgery, it's common to feel a greater sense of self-confidence. And thanks to that renewed feeling, you may see some positive changes in your life. However, body contouring surgery does have its limits. A tighter tummy or bigger breasts may make your figure look more attractive, but it won't necessarily make you more likable or help you get a promotion at work. And if you're basically unhappy, cosmetic surgery won't change that.

Because of this, cosmetic surgeons are careful to weigh your motivation for seeking cosmetic surgery as well as your mental well-being. In general, a surgeon will want to make sure you're seeking

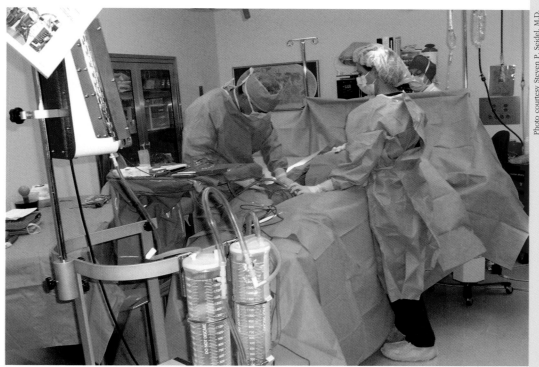

The patient here is undergoing liposuction of the thighs and hips. Liposuction remains one of the most popular cosmetic surgery procedures in the U.S.

body contouring surgery as a way to please yourself, not because your husband or boyfriend is pressuring you to have a procedure. Plus, surgeons will consider you a better candidate if cosmetic surgery is something you've been contemplating for some time as opposed to it being a recent whim. If you're depressed or going through a crisis, such as a divorce, a surgeon may suggest delaying any cosmetic procedures until you feel emotionally stable.

Another key element cosmetic surgeons will take into consideration when evaluating you as a prospective patient is your willingness to take an active role in the experience. Essentially, you should think of yourself

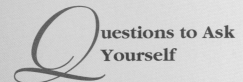

Questions to Ask Yourself

- Are you seeking cosmetic surgery to please yourself or somebody else?

- Are you trying to fix a body flaw or something else in your life?

- Have you exhausted all other efforts to improve your physique, such as diet and exercise?

- Are you willing to listen to your surgeon even if he or she doesn't tell you what you want to hear?

- Do you have any chronic health issues?

- Are your expectations realistic?

- Are you willing to do your part to achieve the best results?

as a partner in the entire process. Cosmetic surgeons consider it your responsibility as a patient to be informed, to ask questions, to communicate your goals, and to follow instructions. As a rule, the more effort you put into the process, the more likely you are to get the results you want.

When Body Contouring Surgery May Not Be for You

Cosmetic surgeons routinely turn down prospective patients for a number of reasons, including unrealistic expectations, a poor attitude, health issues, or detrimental lifestyle habits. If your expectations are unrealistic, you probably won't be pleased with your results even if your final outcome is the best possible. If you're hoping that surgery will change your life or cure your depression, you're setting yourself up for a letdown. And if you aren't willing to make the necessary effort to ensure an excellent result, cosmetic surgeons will urge you to consider other options.

Sometimes, even if your expectations and attitude are on the mark, other health conditions could prevent you from being a good candidate; these conditions include heart, lung, kidney, or liver disease; uncontrollable diabetes; connective-tissue disorders; uncontrolled high blood pressure; autoimmune diseases; and endocrine disorders.

However, having a medical condition doesn't categorically disqualify you for cosmetic surgery. Your surgeon will evaluate your case on an individual basis. As a precaution, you may be required to undergo additional testing or to obtain clearance from a primary-care physician before being accepted as a patient for body contouring.

Other reasons that may make you less than an ideal candidate include being a smoker, being overweight or obese, or having excessive sun exposure. Smoking restricts circulation to the skin, interferes with healing, and accelerates the aging process. All of these can have a negative effect on body contouring procedures. If you're overweight or obese, you may be advised to lose weight before contemplating a body contouring procedure. Excessive sun exposure breaks down collagen and elastin, accelerating the aging process, and contributing to loose skin. Because of loose skin, you may not see optimal results from certain body contouring procedures.

What's the Next Step?

If you think body contouring surgery is right for you, take the time to learn about the various procedures that interest you and make an appointment with an experienced, board-certified plastic surgeon. Only a qualified surgeon can ultimately determine if you qualify for surgery, which procedures would benefit you most, and what kinds of results you can expect. In your quest for a more flattering figure, be prepared to take an active role in the process, which begins with your initial research and continues after you've achieved your new look.

CHAPTER TWO

Choosing a Plastic Surgeon

2

Choosing a Plastic Surgeon

Choosing a surgeon is one of the most important decisions you'll make regarding breast-augmentation and body contouring surgery. To ensure a safe and successful procedure that gives you the results you desire, you'll need to find a highly qualified and experienced plastic surgeon with whom you feel comfortable. Since cosmetic surgery affects your body image, your overall health, *and* your bank account, you should be prepared to spend some quality time on this crucial step.

Begin by asking for referrals from your family physician, gynecologist, dermatologist, friends, and relatives. With the names they give you, do some research of your own. Visit each surgeon's Web site, and call his or her office to ask for more information. By this time, you may have a pretty good feel about one or more of the surgeons so go ahead and schedule an appointment, but take note that some doctors charge a moderate fee for an initial consultation. To zero in on the right surgeon, you need to know what specific qualifications to look for, what to expect from your consultation, what questions to ask, and more.

Surgeon Qualifications

No matter whom you ask or where you turn for advice on choosing a surgeon, you'll be advised to select someone who is well qualified. But as a patient, how do you determine if a surgeon is qualified? When checking into a surgeon's qualifications, the most important things to look for are adequate training, board certification, and experience performing the specific procedure you're considering.

Education and Training

It takes years of specialized training to become a plastic surgeon. First, a surgeon must graduate from college and then successfully complete an additional four years in an accredited medical school. An accredited school is one that meets standards set by a national authority for medical education programs.

Becoming a plastic surgeon requires several years of additional training beyond medical school. The doctor must complete a minimum of five to six years of training in a hospital, where he or she performs surgery under the guidance and supervision of senior-level surgeons. This training period is called a residency. The first few years of the residency usually focus on general surgery, and the last years concentrate on plastic surgery in particular. As the residency progresses, the surgeon's responsibilities increase until he or she is capable of assuming complete responsibility for the surgical care of patients.

By the time a doctor goes into practice as a plastic surgeon, he or she has had plenty of hands-on experience working side by side with senior-level surgeons. But a surgeon's training doesn't end there. Plastic surgeons are required to take continuing medical-education courses throughout their careers in order to keep their certification up to date.

Importance of Board Certification

You've probably heard that it's important to choose a surgeon who is "board-certified." But what exactly does that mean? Being board-certified means that a plastic surgeon has participated in a residency program in both general surgery and plastic surgery and has passed comprehensive written and oral exams. Once a plastic surgeon passes the written and oral exams, board certification is granted. Any surgeon you consider should be certified by the American Board of Plastic Surgery (ABPS). This is the only medical board recognized by the American Board of Medical Specialties (ABMS) that offers certification to surgeons specializing in plastic surgery. It's important to note that there is

> "It's important to choose a plastic surgeon who is board-certified. Also, make sure you have seen before-after photos of patients who had the same procedure you're considering."
>
> —Thomas B. McNemar, M.D.

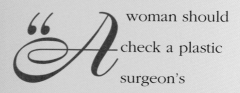

A woman should check a plastic surgeon's credentials. She should also have a good "chemistry" with the surgeon. Consulting with more than one surgeon is perfectly acceptable."

— Steven P. Seidel, M.D.

currently no medical board recognized by the ABMS offering certification in cosmetic surgery.

Plastic surgeons who have earned board certification are required to be recertified every ten years. To qualify for recertification, surgeons must receive additional training on a regular basis. This is often achieved by participating in continuing medical education. In addition, surgeons must continually meet the moral and ethical standards set by the ABPS.

You may be surprised to discover that board certification is a completely voluntary process. It's true, surgeons aren't required to be certified to perform plastic surgery. However, choosing a plastic surgeon who meets rigorous standards set by an authoritative board may give you some peace of mind. To verify a surgeon's certification, go to the ABMS Web site at www.abms.org.

Although board certification is voluntary, having a license to practice medicine is mandatory. In order to legally practice medicine in your state, a surgeon must have a current medical license issued by the state's medical licensing board. You can check with your state's medical board for license verification.

As a final note, beware that many states allow any licensed physician to legally perform cosmetic surgery even though they are not trained plastic surgeons. For your health and to ensure a good result, it's imperative to make sure your doctor is indeed a trained plastic surgeon.

Experience of the Plastic Surgeon

While board certification provides an assurance of training and experience in plastic surgery, you also want to make sure that the doctor you select has ample experience with the procedure you're considering. First, you should look for a plastic surgeon who specializes in cosmetic surgery.

What's the difference between plastic surgery and cosmetic surgery? One way to look at it is that all cosmetic surgery is considered plastic surgery, but not all plastic surgery is considered cosmetic surgery. Plastic surgery encompasses both reconstructive surgery and cosmetic surgery.

Reconstructive surgery refers to operations that are medically necessary to restore normal function or appearance to abnormal structures of the body. Cosmetic surgery, on the other hand, focuses on elective procedures that are performed primarily to reshape and enhance the appearance of normal features of the body. If you're seeking a cosmetic procedure, such as breast augmentation, liposuction, or a tummy tuck, you'd be wise to narrow your search to plastic surgeons who specialize in cosmetic surgery.

When researching cosmetic surgeons, you should find out more about their experience level with the specific procedure you're considering. You may have heard that a good way to gauge a surgeon's expertise is to ask how many years he or she has been performing the procedure you're considering or how many times per year they perform that particular procedure. But how do you know what the "right" number is?

Unfortunately, there is no right answer to this. However, as a rule of thumb, you should look for a surgeon who performs breast augmentation or your desired body contouring procedure at least a few times a month.

Your Consultation

Prior to any surgical procedure, you will have at least one and perhaps two consultations at the doctor's office. This meeting will help you decide if a surgeon is right for you. From the moment you walk into the office, take note of how you are treated. Does the staff greet you pleasantly? Do they respond to your questions? Do you see the doctor promptly? Does the doctor listen to your goals and concerns? The way you are treated at this initial meeting is often a preview of how you will be treated throughout your procedure, so pay attention. Your consultation should include information on the following.

- Pre- and postoperative instructions, including follow-up visits

- Goals clarification

- Surgical techniques and incision sites

- Length of procedure
- Type of anesthesia to be used
- Surgical-center information
- Common side effects, risks, and complications
- Costs

Ask Questions

Going into a consultation well prepared is the best way to ensure that you will get the most out of it. Before your appointment, educate yourself about the specific procedure or procedures you are considering. Make a list of questions to ask the surgeon and be prepared to speak very frankly about what you would like to change about your body. Talking about what makes you self-conscious may be difficult, but by communicating openly, you will be more likely to get the results you desire. By the same token, you need to be willing to listen to what your doctor has to say. You may think you know exactly what procedure you want, but your surgeon may suggest a different procedure as a better way to achieve your goals. Or you may learn about procedures or techniques you didn't know were available. Go to your consultation with an open mind, and you will come out of it a better-informed patient.

Remembering all the details in the days following your consultation can be difficult. Some patients choose to take notes to help them recall the specifics; others bring a friend or relative along to take notes or simply to provide moral support.

Medical History

Before meeting with the doctor, you will most likely be asked to complete a medical-history form. Don't rely solely on your memory to complete these forms because most of us can't recall off the top of our heads the exact date we had our wisdom teeth pulled, the last time we had blood work done, or the address and phone number of our primary physician. If you don't already have copies of your medical records, you may want to get them prior to your appointment and review them. Or simply call your doctor's office to ask for the dates and results of key procedures or lab tests. Most likely, your surgeon won't need to see copies of your medical records, but you may want to check with the surgeon's office prior to your appointment.

Key information you should be prepared to disclose includes:

- Past or current medical conditions

- Hospitalizations

- All previous surgeries

- Allergy and asthma details

- Drugs you're taking (prescription, over-the-counter, vitamins, herbs, supplements, even illegal drugs)

Don't leave anything out of your history because you think it's not important, you're embarrassed about it, or you think it might disqualify you for surgery. If you conceal any health-related information, you could be putting yourself at unnecessary risk. One of the main things surgeons look for in a medical history is smoking. Smoking can affect the circulation in the skin and your ability to heal properly, especially for procedures such as a breast lift and a tummy tuck, so be sure to tell your surgeon if you smoke. Even if you smoke only once in a while, it's important to share this information. Your surgeon may insist that you stop smoking for a certain amount of time prior to your procedure.

Physical Exam

At some point during your consultation, your doctor will perform a physical exam. If you're considering breast augmentation, the surgeon will be looking at the amount of your existing breast tissue, the symmetry of your breasts, nipple placement, and more. If you're a body contouring patient, you can expect the doctor to check for excess fat deposits and loose skin on your abdomen, hips, and thighs, among other areas.

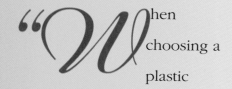

"When choosing a plastic surgeon it is important to choose one with whom you have a good rapport. Part of your surgeon's role is to provide education and be compassionate."

—C. Andrew Salzberg, M.D.

Based on your current appearance, your surgeon can zero in on the specific procedures and techniques that are right for you. After this exam, your surgeon should be able to give you a good idea of the results you can expect. The doctor may recommend additional procedures to help you reach your goal. For example, you may be interested in liposuction, but after an examination of your abdomen, your doctor may suggest that you would benefit more from a tummy tuck in addition to liposuction.

If you're considering breast augmentation, you may discover that combining the procedure with a breast lift would dramatically improve your appearance. A skilled and ethical surgeon will make these suggestions only if they will help you achieve the results you desire and for no other reason. Although cosmetic surgery has been proven to be safe and effective, no surgery is completely risk-free, and no reputable surgeon would suggest additional surgeries that could put you at unnecessary risk.

For various reasons, the doctor may recommend that you wait for some time before undergoing surgery. Or you may discover that your ultimate goal isn't within reach. Even so, your surgeon may make recommendations for a procedure that will make a marked improvement in your appearance.

View Before-and-After Photos

Some surgeons will show you before-and-after photos of former patients as a way to illustrate the kinds of results that can be achieved. Of course, doctors want to present their best work, but the images you see should represent a variety of results, including some that aren't perfect. For example, if you are considering breast augmentation, be wary of a doctor who shows you only photos of patients who look like *Playboy* models. Likewise, potential tummy-tuck patients should check that the photos they see show visible scars. No surgeon can make an invisible tummy-tuck scar—if you don't see a scar, the photos may have been altered. To get a better idea of what your individual results might look like, ask your doctor to show you images of patients with the same body type and similar concerns you have.

In addition to judging the quality of the doctor's work, use this opportunity to express what you're hoping to achieve. For instance, if you're reviewing photos of breast augmentation patients, tell the surgeon, "these are too big," "these are too small," or "I'd like something close to this size." This will help you communicate your goals and improve your chances of getting the results you want.

View Computer Imaging

Some surgeons are taking a high-tech approach involving computer imaging to give you an estimate of your postoperative appearance. With this technique, someone in the doctor's office will take digital photos of you, which may include a frontal, side profile, forty-five-degree angle, or backside view, depending on the procedure you're considering. The photos are then downloaded into a computer. Using digital-imaging software, your surgeon can alter your photos to reveal what certain procedures might do for you.

For example, to give you an idea of what you might expect from breast augmentation, the surgeon can add curves to frontal, side, and forty-five-degree-angle views. If you're considering liposuction of your hips and thighs, your surgeon can reshape them right before your eyes, giving you a glimpse of your anticipated silhouette as seen from the front, the side, and the back. Using frontal and side-profile views, your surgeon can "sculpt" your abdomen on screen to reveal what you realistically can expect from a tummy tuck.

When viewing your own before-and-after images, use this opportunity to communicate what you would like to change about your body and if you like what you see in the "after" image. This will ensure that you and your surgeon are on the same page in terms of what can be achieved for you.

Beware that there are some potential drawbacks to computer imaging. A computer can't take into account your skin tone, your healing ability, or your overall health. That means the image you see on screen is

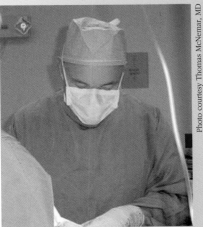

Photo courtesy Thomas McNemar, MD

When choosing a plastic surgeon, make sure the surgeon is experienced in performing the procedure you wish to have.

> *Your surgery should be done in a certified surgical center. This gives you reassurance that safety guidelines are in place.*
>
> —Thomas B. McNemar, M.D.

no guarantee of what the future holds for you. For this reason, you should view computer imaging simply as a general idea of what to expect.

Talk to Former Patients

One of the best ways to determine if a surgeon is right for you is to talk to former patients who have had the same procedure you're considering. Most surgeons have contact information for patients who have agreed to speak about their experiences. Be sure to talk to at least one patient who experienced a complication or who needed revisional surgery to see how the surgeon's office handles these issues.

Questions to Ask a Former Patient

- Did you feel comfortable with the surgeon and staff?
- Did the surgeon spend enough time with you and answer all your questions?
- Did you feel rushed?
- Did you have any problems after surgery, no matter how minor?
- How did the surgeon and staff respond to your problems?
- On follow-up visits, did you see the surgeon or just a nurse?
- Did the surgeon's office call and check on you following your surgery?
- Were your phone calls returned promptly?
- Were you pleased with your results?
- Would you go back to the surgeon for another procedure?

Is the Surgical Center Accredited?

Most likely, your procedure will be performed in an office-based surgical suite or an outpatient-surgery facility rather than in a hospital. No matter where your surgery takes place, you want to make sure that the facility is accredited, which means it meets nationally recognized standards for safety and quality.

Any surgery facility you're considering should be certified by one of the nation's three main accrediting organizations: the American Association for the Accreditation of Ambulatory Surgery Facilities, the Accreditation Association for Ambulatory Health Care, or the Joint Commission on Accreditation of Healthcare Organizations. (See the Resources section for more information on these organizations.) Accredited facilities are reviewed and inspected on a regular basis and must meet stringent requirements for surgeon credentials, equipment, operating-room safety, and personnel.

Because of these high standards, there's an excellent safety record associated with plastic-surgery procedures performed by board-certified plastic surgeons in accredited surgical facilities. According to a 1997 study, published in *Plastic and Reconstructive Surgery*, the journal of the American Society of Plastic Surgeons, the rate of serious complications for procedures performed in accredited facilities was less than one-half of 1 percent.

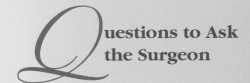

Questions to Ask the Surgeon

- Are you board-certified?

- What procedure or procedures do you recommend for me?

- What are the risks and potential complications?

- What results can I expect?

- What do I need to do to ensure optimal results?

- Will I have to take time off from work? How long?

- When can I resume normal activities?

- Will I require additional surgeries throughout my lifetime?

- Who will be assisting you with the surgery and what are their credentials?

- Is the surgical facility accredited?

- Are you or a nurse available for questions?

CHAPTER THREE

Body Contouring Surgery: What to Expect

3

Body Contouring Surgery: What to Expect

If you've ever tuned in to one of the many cosmetic-surgery-makeover shows on TV, you might think you know what to expect from cosmetic surgery. But there's much more to the surgery experience than what you see in a one-hour television episode. Your journey begins long before you ever set foot in the operating room and continues throughout the weeks and months following your procedure. The way you treat yourself before and after surgery can greatly affect the safety and success of your procedure as well as the speed of your recovery. Whether you're considering breast augmentation, liposuction, or a tummy tuck, your surgeon will be counting on you to take an active role in the process.

By understanding what to expect throughout the surgery experience, you can make the wisest choices to ensure the best possible outcome for your body contouring procedure.

Preparing for Your Surgery

At a preoperative visit or consultation, your doctor will provide you with detailed instructions that spell out what you need to do before surgery. These instructions are based on your surgeon's experience and expertise and are intended to promote safety and healing. Following these directions will greatly improve your chances of a safe and successful procedure and a smooth recovery. Call your surgeon's office and ask about instructions you don't understand.

Arrange for a Caregiver

You'll need to have someone drive you to and from surgery and care for you for at least the first twenty-four hours after surgery. Why can't you drive yourself? Surgeons often prescribe a mild sedative the night before surgery to make sure you get a good night's sleep, and driving is not advised for forty-eight hours after taking a sedative. And following your surgery, you can expect to feel sleepy or groggy from the anesthesia, so you won't be able to drive a car safely.

Having a responsible adult care for you for at least the first day following surgery is extremely important. On your first day at home, you can expect to feel sleepy and have some pain or discomfort, depending on the type of surgical procedure you had. To avoid unnecessary swelling or bleeding, your surgeon will instruct you to restrict your movement, including no bending, straining, or exercise. As a result, you may need assistance with simple, everyday tasks such as going to the bathroom or preparing a meal. In addition, if you have a medical emergency, it's imperative that someone is available to call for help or drive you to the hospital or surgeon's office if necessary. For these reasons, you must have someone at home to care for you.

Stop Taking Certain Medications

Your doctor will advise you to stop taking certain medications for a specific amount of time prior to surgery. Some prescription medications, over-the-counter remedies, vitamins, herbs, and supplements that are perfectly safe to take on a normal basis may not be advisable when you're scheduled for surgery or anesthesia. Specifically, anything that thins the blood and prevents it from clotting normally is off-limits because it increases your chances of blood loss during the operation. This includes prescription blood thinners, such as heparin or coumadin, any over-the-counter pain relievers containing aspirin or ibuprofen, and vitamin E supplements. Your surgeon will provide you with a list of substances to avoid and will indicate how far in advance of your surgery to stop taking them. If you're taking something that isn't on the list, don't assume it's okay. Ask your doctor about it.

On the flip side, you may be asked to start taking a daily multivitamin to promote general health and vitamin C to promote healing. In some instances, iron pills may be recommended to help produce red blood cells.

Stop Drinking Alcohol

In addition to avoiding certain medications, you will be instructed to refrain from drinking alcoholic beverages for approximately one to two weeks prior to surgery because they can also thin the blood.

Fill Your Prescriptions

Prior to your procedure, the surgeon will generally give you prescriptions for pain medication, antibiotics, antinausea medication, and perhaps surgical soap. Even though you may not need to use some of these until after you've had surgery, it's important to fill the prescriptions beforehand. Even if you have a high tolerance for pain or an "iron stomach" and aren't sure you'll need the pain or antinausea medication, it's better to have it on hand just in case. Remember that you will be in no condition to drive to or stand in line at a pharmacy following surgery. The last thing you want is to arrive home or wake up in the middle of the night in pain or nauseated and not have your medication available.

Quit Smoking

If you're a smoker, you must be willing to stop smoking for a prescribed amount of time prior to surgery and throughout your recovery. Depending on the body contouring procedure you've chosen and your surgeon's advice, you may be asked to quit for as little as one week or for more than a month before your procedure.

Why is smoking so detrimental to surgery? Smoking constricts the small blood vessels near the skin surface, which decreases a person's skin circulation. You don't have to be a heavy smoker to restrict skin circulation; even smoking a single cigarette can constrict the small blood vessels for as much as ninety minutes. These same blood vessels are also affected when a surgeon makes an incision in the skin, which means the skin circulation is further compromised.

When blood supply to the skin is decreased in this manner, it can interfere with wound healing and lead to infection or skin death, or necrosis. In fact, it is estimated that smokers experience skin death three to six times more often than nonsmokers. The larger the incisions your procedure involves, the greater the risk. For example, tummy tucks involve incisions that are much larger than those used in liposuction or breast augmentation procedures. Therefore, smokers who undergo a tummy tuck are more at risk than those who choose liposuction or breast augmentation.

Schedule Lab Tests

Depending on your medical condition and your age, you may need to undergo certain lab tests prior to surgery. The results of these tests will help your doctor decide if you are healthy enough to undergo the procedure.

- *Complete blood count (CBC)*: To check for abnormalities in the blood, a surgeon will commonly order a complete blood count, often referred to as a CBC. A CBC measures thirteen blood levels, including three that are very important to the success of any surgery: white blood cells, platelets, and hemoglobin. If you don't have enough white blood cells, your body may not be able to fight

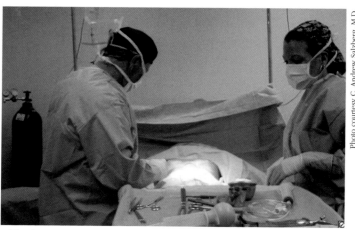

Photo courtesy C. Andrew Salzberg, M.D.

The breast augmentation procedure underway here will take approximately an hour and a half. The patient is receiving IV sedation.

infections that can occur following surgery. If your platelet levels are too low, you're more at risk for excessive bleeding and bruising. A deficiency of hemoglobin, which carries oxygen to your body's organs and tissues, can lead to poor or delayed healing.

- *Electrocardiogram (ECG or EKG):* An electro-cardiogram measures the electrical activity of the heart. Electrodes are attached to your chest. With each heartbeat, an electrical current is transmitted through the electrodes to the EKG machine, which then prints out a report for your physician. The main things your surgeon will look for in this report are any irregularities in the heartbeat and any evidence of past heart attacks. Based on this information, a physician can determine if your heart is strong enough to handle the stress of surgery and anesthesia.

- *Chest X-ray:* A basic chest X-ray is an important tool that can reveal problems with the lungs, respiratory tract, heart, or lymph glands. In particular, your doctor will be looking for any signs of heart disease, such as congenital heart disease or heart failure, or lung conditions, such as emphysema or fluid in the lungs. If any heart or lung abnormalities are present, additional testing will likely be necessary.

- *Mammogram:* A mammogram is an X-ray of the breast that is used to detect breast cancer and other forms of breast disease. It is recommended that women who are forty years of age or older get a mammogram every year. During a mammogram, a technician positions and compresses each breast between two plates before taking the X-ray views. Breast compression may cause some discomfort.

Plastic surgeons often recommend that patients who are forty or over get a mammogram prior to breast augmentation for two reasons. First, if any evidence of breast cancer is detected, a surgeon will not perform breast augmen- tation. (In some instances, breast augmentation may be performed after breast cancer has been treated.) Second, a preaug-mentation mam- mogram can pro- vide a baseline that can be compared with future mam- mograms of your breasts with implants.

Plan for Your Recovery

Prior to surgery, you may also want to think about ways to make your recovery more enjoyable and stress-free. A well-planned recovery period can speed healing, relieve boredom, and keep your spirits high. Go grocery shopping before your surgery and prepare a few meals in advance. Do any necessary housekeeping or laundry before the day of your operation so you won't feel guilty about clothes piling up or dust accumulating while you recover. Stock up on a few good books, favorite magazines, or DVDs. Entertaining diversions can make your recovery a more pleasant experience.

Follow Your Diet Instructions

You will probably be instructed not to eat or drink anything after midnight before your surgery

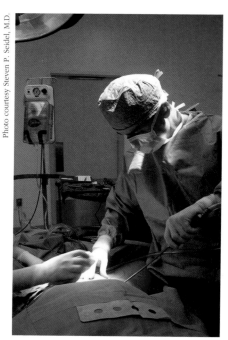

Photo courtesy Steven P. Seidel, M.D.

The liposuction patient here is receiving twilight sedation, the anesthesia commonly used for liposuction.

except for the few sips of water needed to swallow your medication. Why do you need to fast? The administration of anesthesia can induce vomiting. If your stomach is empty, this isn't a problem. But if it occurs when you have food or drink in your stomach, it can lead to serious consequences. As mentioned earlier, you should stop drinking alcohol a week or two before your surgery because alcohol tends to thin the blood and can lead to increased bruising.

Shower Instructions

It's important to cleanse the surgical site with a prescription surgical soap or antibacterial soap of your doctor's choosing the night before and the morning of your procedure. You will probably be asked to scrub a wide area surrounding the surgical site for up to ten minutes at night and again the following morning. Cleaning the area in this manner will decrease the number of bacteria in your skin and

will minimize the chances of developing an infection after surgery. After showering, don't apply any moisturizers, skin conditioners, makeup, or deodorant unless your doctor says it's okay. Fragrances may also be off-limits.

What to Wear to the Surgery Center

You can greatly increase your comfort level after surgery by wearing loose-fitting clothing that doesn't pull over your head. For example, it's better to wear a shirt, sweater, or sweatshirt that buttons or zips up the front. Since you may be asked to refrain from bending over after surgery, wear shoes that you can slide into. Because some body contouring procedures may cause some fluid drainage following surgery, you may want to wear something old so you won't be upset if it gets dirty or stained.

What to Leave at Home

It's best to leave all valuables at home. You'll be asked to remove hairpins, wigs, and jewelry, including wedding rings and watches. You'll also be asked to take out your contact lenses if you wear them, so you may prefer to leave them at home and wear eyeglasses instead.

Arriving at the Surgery Center

Knowing what to expect when you reach the surgical center can help minimize stress on a day when you're likely to be feeling anxious. Once you arrive at the surgical center, you'll most likely be asked to leave your personal items (purse, glasses, etc.) with either your caregiver or in a designated area. The surgeon and staff will then prepare you for your body contouring procedure. The staff will have you change into a hospital gown and may also supply you with a hairnet and socks or protective booties to wear. You also may have a brief meeting with the surgeon to discuss any last-minute questions or postoperative instructions. Your surgeon will use a special surgical marking pen to draw on your body to indicate the placement of the incision(s). To help you relax, you may be given a sedative by pill or injection. If you're not given a sedative and you are feeling anxious, ask for one.

Monitoring pads may be taped to your chest to keep track of your vital signs, including your temperature, heart rate, oxygen levels, blood pressure, and breathing. The staff will start an IV in your arm to administer anesthetics, antibiotics, and other medications. When the IV needle is inserted, you will feel a slight stinging for a few seconds.

Undergoing Surgery

The length of your surgery depends on the procedure you're having, the techniques being used, and your surgeon. Two surgeons performing the same operation using the same techniques may take very different amounts of time to finish the procedure. Ask your surgeon approximately how long you are expected to be in the operating room.

Your surgeon isn't alone in the operating room. The surgical team may include a physician anesthesiologist or certified registered nurse anesthetist, a registered nurse, and a trained operating-room technician.

Anesthesia

Your cosmetic-surgery procedure will require some form of anesthesia in order to keep you pain-free during the operation. Like many patients, you may feel some anxiety about being "put under" during your procedure. Although these feelings are common, you should know that anesthesia is safer than ever, thanks to new drugs and major advances in monitoring equipment. To ensure your safety, anesthesia should be administered by a physician anesthesiologist or a certified registered nurse anesthetist.

There are three types of anesthesia that may be used for your cosmetic surgery procedure. The one your surgeon chooses depends on the procedure you're having, your physical condition, and your reactions to medications.

General Anesthesia

General anesthesia renders you unconscious, keeps you pain-free, and blocks your memory of the procedure. With general anesthesia, you're unable to breathe on your own, so the anesthesiologist will place a breathing tube down your windpipe (trachea). General anesthesia agents can stay in your body for up to twenty-four hours after being administered, and you won't feel completely normal until it has been totally eliminated from your system.

Sedation Anesthesia

Also called monitored anesthesia care (MAC) or twilight sedation, sedation anesthesia uses pain relievers and sedatives to minimize discomfort and to induce relaxation and drowsiness. This form of anesthesia can be combined with local anesthetics, which helps control pain. With this method, you will be able to breathe on your own so you won't require a breathing tube. The recovery from sedation anesthesia is rapid, with most patients feeling normal within an hour or two.

Regional Anesthesia

Regional anesthesia blocks pain in a specific region of the body. Example of regional anesthesia are spinals and epidurals, commonly used during childbirth, which numbs the lower half of the body. Regional anesthesia allows you to breathe on your own so a breathing tube isn't necessary. It can be used in conjunction with sedation to make you feel calm and comfortable. When sedation is used with regional anesthesia, the recovery time is usually about an hour or two.

Monitoring during Surgery

Advances in monitoring care during surgery have helped make anesthesia safer than ever. During your surgery, the anesthesiologist will monitor your circulation, oxygen levels, temperature, and breathing.

To monitor your circulation, the anesthesiologist will use a number of methods. An EKG tracks your heart rate and alerts the anesthesiologist to any irregularities in your heartbeat. A blood pressure cuff will signal any rise or drop in your blood pressure. In addition, the anesthesiologist will listen to your heart and take your pulse manually.

To measure the amount of oxygen in your blood, a small device called a pulse oximeter is placed on your fingertip. Any drop in your oxygen levels sets off an alarm.

Your temperature will be watched closely to avoid a drop in body temperature.

If a breathing tube is required, a monitor allows the anesthesiologist to verify that the tube is properly placed and that your ventilation level is adequate.

After Your Procedure
In the Recovery Room

After your surgery, you will be moved to the recovery room. Here, you may be given extra oxygen, and your vital signs will continue to be monitored. The surgical staff will also be checking for any bleeding, breathing problems, or a reaction to anesthesia. Most patients are ready to go home one to four hours following surgery, but you may need to stay overnight depending on your procedure. Under no circumstances will you be allowed to drive after surgery, so be sure you've arranged for a driver and at-home caregiver as detailed in your preoperative instructions.

Side Effects of Anesthesia

Anesthesia is associated with certain side effects. Following anesthesia, you can expect to feel groggy and fatigued. Anesthesia can also cause nausea or vomiting. Fortunately, improvements in the drugs and techniques used have made nausea and vomiting far less common. If you feel nauseated, let the surgical

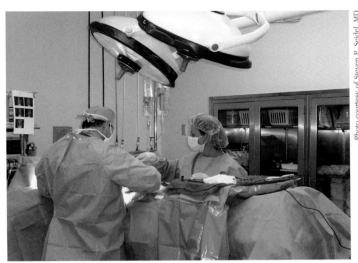

Breast augmentation surgery, underway here, ranks among the five most popular cosmetic surgery procedures among women.

staff know right away, and you'll be given antinausea medication.

It is also possible to have an allergic reaction to anesthesia, although this is usually preventable. When your doctor reviews your medical history, he or she will be looking for any possible allergies and will make choices regarding anesthesia accordingly. In the unlikely event of a reaction, you will probably be monitored and treated in the recovery room.

Side Effects of Surgery

There are potential side effects and risks associated with every surgery, including body-contouring procedures. Side effects are considered normal and are usually temporary in nature. However, complications aren't normal and require immediate medical attention.

Side effects associated with any body contouring procedure include pain, swelling, bruising, and temporary numbness in the treated area. For more details about these symptoms as they relate to specific body contouring procedures, see the individual chapters on breast augmentation, liposuction, and tummy tucks.

Scars are a permanent side effect of any surgery. Scars go through a maturation process. At first, a new scar may feel firm and is pink, red or purple. As time progresses, your body will remodel the scar and it will feel softer, become flat and the color will fade to your normal skin color. This scar maturation process, however, will take at least 6 months and up to one to two years.

One common aftereffect of cosmetic surgery that you may not anticipate is a brief emotional letdown or depression. Don't be alarmed if you feel a little down in the days following your surgery. It's common to question your decision to have surgery when your body is swollen, bruised, and aching. These feelings often surface about three days after surgery, at a time when your energy levels have improved but your appearance hasn't. The emotional low may stem from metabolic changes in the body, fatigue, stress, or the frustration felt when results don't appear as quickly as hoped.

Knowing that a postoperative letdown is a natural phase of the healing process may help you cope with it better. Following your doctor's instructions is one of the best things you can do to help keep these feelings to a minimum because the faster you heal and the sooner you get back to normal activities, the better you'll feel.

Risks of Cosmetic Surgery

The risks of complications involved with body contouring surgery are real, and it's important to understand them. The following list includes risks associated with any body contouring procedure.

- *Infection*: Thanks to the antibiotics used in the operating room and during recovery, infections aren't common with body contouring procedures. Superficial infections may be treated with oral antibiotics; deeper infections often require intravenous antibiotics or surgical drainage.

- *Anesthesia reaction*: Allergic reactions to anesthesia and other medications are usually preventable. When your doctor reviews your medical history, he or she will be looking for any possible allergies and will make choices regarding anesthesia accordingly. In the unlikely event of a reaction, you will probably be monitored and treated in the recovery room.

- *Postoperative bleeding*: Any postoperative bleeding should be minimal and should stop completely within a few days. Any excessive bleeding should be reported to your doctor.

- *Hematoma*: When blood collects under the incision, it is called a hematoma. If a hematoma forms, it is usually within the first 24 hours after surgery. Symptoms may include swelling, pain, and bruising. Your surgeon needs to know about a hematoma, since it might indicate ongoing bleeding. Also, leaving the pooled blood in place can increase the risk of infection. In order to drain a hematoma, the surgeon numbs the skin with a local anesthetic and opens the incision enough to drain the hematoma and control any bleeding. Then, the incision is closed. If the hematoma is small, the procedure may be performed in the surgeon's office, but if the hematoma is large, the surgeon may choose to perform the procedure in the operating room.

- *Seroma*: When serum, the clear liquid portion of the blood, accumulates near the incision, it's called a seroma. The body can usually absorb a small seroma, but if it is large, it may need to be drained through the use of drainage tubes. Seromas usually form later, days after the surgery.

- *Incision complications*: In some instances, incisions may separate. These wounds usually heal with minor treatment by the surgeon and don't require additional surgery, but they may prolong the healing process. Smokers are more at risk for incision complications.

- *Keloid and hypertrophic scars*: In any surgery, there is a possibility of developing unsightly scars that are thick, raised, and pigmented. Keloid scars form large mounds of scar tissue that go beyond the boundaries of the incision. Hypertrophic scars look similar to keloid scars but usually don't get as big and may fade over time. Your doctor may try a variety of nonsurgical techniques to help the scar flatten and fade evenly. If these attempts don't work, your surgeon may suggest cutting away the scar and restitching the incision, cryosurgery, or steroid injections.

- *Tissue necrosis*: When blood supply to the skin is compromised, or an infection gets out of control, it can lead to tissue necrosis, also called skin death. Tissue necrosis generally occurs at incision sites and is more common with larger incisions, such as those associated with tummy tucks. Smokers are more at risk for skin death since smoking compromises skin circulation. In the early stages of necrosis, tissue may appear blue, purple, or gray and may be painful. In advanced stages, tissue turns gray or black and may smell or become infected. In minor cases, the skin may be allowed to heal on its own. Treatment for more severe cases may include tissue removal and hyperbaric oxygen therapy, a form of wound treatment in which oxygen is provided in a concealed chamber.

Post-Surgical Instructions

To speed healing and make your recovery more comfortable, your doctor will give you detailed postoperative instructions. Following these instructions will help you get back in the swing of things as soon as possible. Make sure your caregiver is also aware of the instructions since the effects of surgery and anesthesia may prevent you from remembering all the details. The following instructions apply to any body contouring procedure.

- Drink plenty of fluids. Even if you don't have much of an appetite, which is normal, your body needs fluids.

- If you feel nauseated, drink carbonated sodas and eat crackers to settle your stomach. If your stomach feels okay, start with a bland diet and progress to your normal diet.

- Don't drink any alcohol for about ten days because it can dilate the blood vessels and increase postoperative bleeding. Also avoid alcohol while taking pain medication or sedatives as this can be a dangerous combination.

- Avoid smoking and secondhand smoke for up to thirty days after surgery.

- Protect the surgical areas from impact or trauma during your recovery.

- Protect your scars from the sun for up to a year by wearing sunscreen. Sunlight can interfere with the proper fading of scars.

Pain Management

To ease your comfort during the recovery period, your surgeon will make recommendations for pain management. The degree of pain experienced following body contouring surgery is highly individual and can range from mild to severe. Depending on

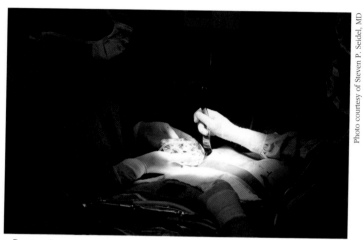

During breast augmentation surgery, the surgeon inserts a partially-filled saline implant through an incision in the inframammary fold. The implant will be fully inflated after insertion.

your procedure, your pain-relief options may include opioid and nonopioid medications.

Opioid Medications

Opioid pain relievers, also called opiates or narcotics, require a prescription from your surgeon. These drugs can be effective in relieving moderate to severe pain by inhibiting the transmission of pain messages to the brain. Side effects associated with opioids include sleepiness, slowed breathing, nausea, and constipation. If you experience any side effects, inform your surgeon and he or she may prescribe another medication.

After body contouring surgery, commonly prescribed narcotic medications include:

- Lortab
- Percocet
- Darvocet
- Mepergan fortis

The medication, Mepergan fortis, contains a narcotic, and it also contains the drug phenergan, which combats nausea. For optimal pain management, your surgeon will likely suggest that you "stay ahead" of any pain by taking the pain medications as directed, rather than waiting to take the pills after pain has begun.

Opioids are also known to produce feelings of euphoria, which is why they are sometimes abused. If you're concerned about becoming addicted to prescription pain pills, your fears are unfounded. Cosmetic surgeons stress that taking these drugs as directed for a short period of time following surgery will not lead to addiction.

Nonopioid Medication

Nonopioid pain relievers are not opiates or narcotics, and many do not require a prescription from your doctor. These medications include acetaminophen and nonsteroidal anti-inflammatory drugs (NSAIDs), such as ibuprofen or naproxen. Acetaminophen is found in Tylenol; ibuprofen is a component of Advil and Motrin; and naproxen is the active ingredient in Aleve. Acetaminophen and NSAIDs relieve mild to moderate pain, with NSAIDs offering added relief from inflammation. Side effects are rarely associated with acetaminophen when taken for a few days or a few weeks. NSAIDs can cause stomach pain, heartburn, constipation, and dizziness.

In the Weeks Ahead

As the healing process continues in the weeks ahead, you'll feel more energized and you'll begin returning to normal activities. Ask your doctor for a specific timetable for resuming activities, such as:

- Driving a car
- Returning to office work
- Resuming light housework
- Resuming nonstrenuous activities
- Resuming sexual activity
- Resuming strenuous physical activities and housework
- Going swimming

Questions to Ask Your Surgeon

- Are there any medications, vitamins, or supplements I should avoid?
- What kind of anesthesia will be used?
- What are some of the common side effects associated with cosmetic surgery?
- Will I need pain medication?
- What do I need to do following surgery to ensure a speedy recovery?
- When will I be able to return to normal activities?

CHAPTER FOUR

Your Breast Augmentation Procedure

4

Your Breast Augmentation Procedure

*D*o you wish your breasts were bigger? Would you love to fill out a sweater, or wear a plunging neckline without being embarrassed about your lack of cleavage? If you've ever felt self-conscious about the size or shape of your breasts, you may want to consider breast augmentation.

This highly sought-after procedure is becoming increasingly popular—since 1997, the number of women choosing to undergo the procedure has more than tripled to nearly 350,000 per year. Considering that cultural acceptance of augmentation is at an all-time high and that clinical studies have alleviated safety concerns about saline implants, it's no surprise that so many women are contemplating the procedure. And we aren't just talking about women who want to be swimsuit models. Women of all ages and from every profession imaginable are opting to enhance their breasts with implants.

Are You a Candidate for Breast Augmentation?

If you would like your breasts to look fuller and more shapely, you may be a candidate for breast augmentation. Do you think your breasts are too small or not in proportion with the rest of your body? You may benefit from the procedure. If your breasts have lost their original shape or firmness due to pregnancy, breast-feeding, or menopause, you may see improvements with augmentation. The procedure can also help correct breasts that differ in size or shape. And it can benefit women who feel self-conscious about having odd-shaped breasts, such as tuberous breasts, a condition in which the breasts have a long, narrow mound of breast tissue protruding from the chest wall.

The procedure is performed on women of any age, although many surgeons choose not to operate on anyone under the age of eighteen. The best candidates for breast augmentation are in good overall health and have realistic goals.

When Breast Augmentation May Not Be for You

In some instances, breast augmentation may not be right for you. Doctors will not perform breast augmentation surgery on you if you are pregnant or nursing a baby. And if you plan to become pregnant in the near future, your surgeon may suggest you delay having surgery until a later date. Pregnancy and breast-feeding can cause significant changes in the size, shape, and firmness of your breasts; therefore, if you've had augmentation prior to pregnancy and breast-feeding, you may be unhappy with the way your breasts look after pregnancy or breast-feeding.

If you plan to have children, you should be aware that breast-implant surgery might affect the ability to breast-feed. If breast-feeding is extremely important to you, discuss it with your surgeon. He or she may suggest specific incision sites that are less likely to interfere with breast-feeding or may advise you to wait until after you've had children.

Teenage girls who are considering breast augmentation should realize that many surgeons will not perform the procedure on anyone who has not reached the age of eighteen. Conventional wisdom dictates that a young woman's body may still be maturing during the later teenage years, and it is advisable to wait until the breasts are fully developed before undergoing augmentation. Some surgeons also question the emotional maturity of very young women who may not grasp the long-term consequences of the procedure or who may have

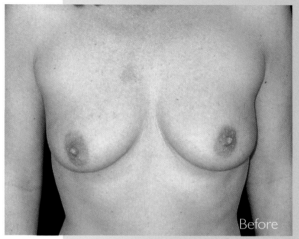

Before

Age: 32. Height: 5' 3"
Weight: 118. Bra size: 36 B

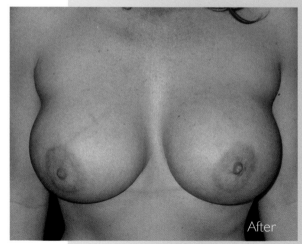

After

Bra size: 36 C. Six weeks postoperative
Incision: inframammary

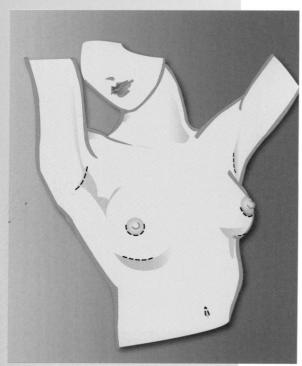

Breast implants may be inserted through incisions in the armpit, around the areola, in the inframammary fold, or though the navel.

questionable motives for wanting the procedure in the first place. There are surgeons who will perform augmentation on younger patients on a case-by-case basis, but generally only with parent approval.

Undergoing Breast Augmentation Surgery

A breast augmentation procedure usually lasts one to two hours. Your surgeon has several choices for the type of incisions to be made for inserting the implants. Once this incision is made, the surgeon will create a "pocket" to accommodate the breast implant beneath the breast tissue, either above or below your chest muscles. He or she will then insert the implant into the pocket, fill it with saline, and position it to achieve the desired effect.

Once the optimal result is attained, your surgeon will close the incision site with sutures. Sutures used in breast augmentation can be either absorbable or nonabsorbable. Absorbable sutures are placed below the skin and, like the name suggests, are absorbed by the body and don't require removal. Nonabsorbable sutures, on the other hand, require removal in your surgeon's office.

Placement of Incisions

Along with your plastic surgeon, you have several options when deciding on the placement of incisions, through which your implants will be inserted. Each of these incision locations has its advantages and disadvantages. Your surgeon will discuss with you which approach is appropriate for you. For most women, it's a matter of preference—where they prefer to have the scars. However, your surgeon may also make recommendations, based on the size and shape of your breasts. To help minimize the length of these scars, many surgeons insert implants when they are empty and fill them during surgery.

Inframammary

The most commonly used approach, an *inframammary* incision is made within the fold or crease under the breast. Of all the incision site options, this one offers the surgeon the best visibility for creating the pocket for the implant. The scar, resulting from this type of incision, is usually not visible when you are standing, but most likely will be visible when you lie down.

Periareolar

A *periareolar* incision is made around the nipple, generally on the lower half or inner edge of the areola, the pigmented skin around the nipple. Many women like the fact that the pigment helps to conceal the scar. However, this incision site is the most likely to interfere with a woman's ability to breast-feed and may also cause loss of sensation in the nipple.

Transaxillary

A *transaxillary* incision is made in the armpit area. Because this incision site is farther away from the actual breast, the surgeon will normally be required to use a probe equipped with a miniature fiber-optic camera to be able to see inside the breast. Although the scar under the arm is visible when the arm is raised, many women prefer this method because it doesn't leave a scar directly on the breast. The transaxillary incision is less likely to interfere with breast-feeding than the periareolar incision.

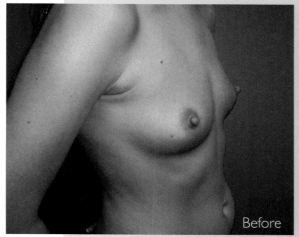

Age: 21. Height: 5' 4"
Weight: 115. Bra size: 32 A

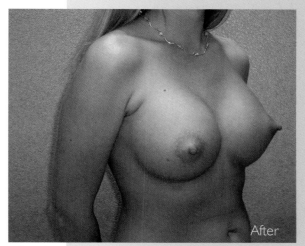

Bra size: 32 C. Six weeks postoperative
Incision: inframammary

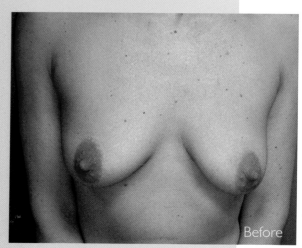

Age: 37. Height: 5' 11"
Weight: 145. Bra size: 36 B

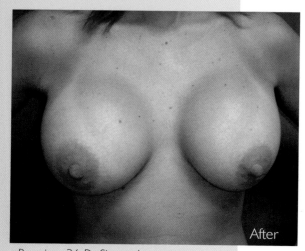

Bra size: 36 D. Six weeks postoperative
Incision: transaxillary

Transumbilical

A *transumbilical* incision is made in the belly button. With this incision, the surgeon uses special equipment to tunnel under the skin to the breast area. Getting the implants positioned for optimal results is considered challenging with this incision, and relatively few surgeons use the transumbilical approach. This approach for implant insertion is also referred to as TUBA—transumbilical breast augmentation.

Types of Implants

Thanks to technological advances, breast implants currently come in a wide variety of sizes, shapes, and surface textures. But what exactly is a breast implant? A breast implant is a sac with a silicone elastomer (rubberlike) outer shell that can be filled with either sterile saline (saltwater) or silicone gel. Some implants are prefilled; others are filled during surgery through a valve in the implant. Remember that no single implant is best for everyone, so talk to your surgeon to determine which one is right for you.

Saline

Saline implants are the only option available to the vast majority of women seeking breast augmentation. Saline implants consist of a silicone elastomer shell, which is filled with sterile saline. The saline solution is very similar to the fluids in the human body, and if a saline implant ruptures or leaks, the fluid is absorbed into the body and eliminated through urination.

Silicone

Silicone implants also have a silicone elastomer shell and are filled with silicone gel. Many surgeons and women alike believe silicone implants feel more natural than saline implants. However, FDA restrictions currently permit the use of silicone-gel implants only in controlled clinical studies for the purposes of reconstruction after mastectomy, correction of congenital deformities, or replacement of ruptured silicone-gel implants that were used for augmentation.

You may recall hearing about the controversy in the 1990s over the safety of silicone implants. Leaks in silicone implants are not easily detected, and some women whose implants ruptured claimed the silicone caused health problems. However, years of studies have produced no hard data linking silicone implants with disease.

Shape of Implants

Round

Round implants are by far the most commonly used in breast augmentation and offer certain advantages over other options. They are less expensive than other shapes, and if they rotate within the breast, there is no visible effect. A variation of the round implant is called a high-profile implant. This implant is round but slightly narrower in width and offers greater projection from the chest wall. Women who have a small frame and narrow chest may benefit from a high-profile implant.

Anatomical

Anatomical implants—also called teardrop, shaped, or contoured implants—are designed to mimic the natural slope of a woman's breasts and are fuller on the bottom than on the top. In some instances, these implants may produce a more natural look. However, studies have shown that anatomical implants placed below the pectoral muscle (submuscular) may lose their teardrop shape and assume a round shape. Anatomical implants can also rotate within the breast, causing an abnormal shape. You can expect to pay more if you decide to go with anatomical implants.

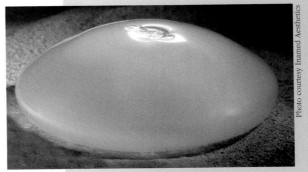

Photo courtesy Inamed Aesthetics

The most commonly used implants are round, smooth implants.

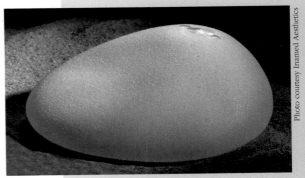

Photo courtesy Inamed Aesthetics

Textured, anatomical implants are an alternative to round implants.

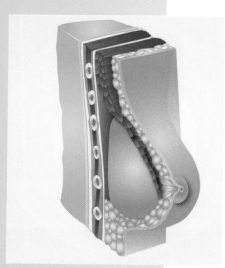

The implant placement is submuscular, under the pectoral muscle.

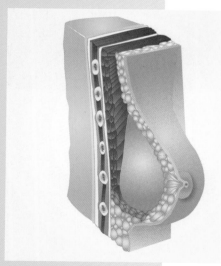

This implant placement is subglandular, above the pectoral muscle.

Texture of Implants

Smooth

The vast majority of women choose implants that have a smooth surface. With a smooth surface, the implant is less likely to develop visible wrinkling, or rippling, a complication associated with augmentation. On the other hand, smooth implants are more prone to shifting position within the breast.

Textured

Textured implants have a rough outer shell. These implants were introduced as a way to reduce capsular contracture, a complication associated with augmentation, in which scar tissue forms around the implant. However, large-scale studies have shown no difference in the likelihood of developing capsular contracture with either smooth or textured implants. Textured implants are more often associated with visible wrinkling, but are less likely to shift within the breast.

Placement of Implants

Submuscular

Submuscular placement of implants means they are placed partially below the pectoral muscle. The upper portion of the implant is placed under the muscle while the lower portion lies below the breast tissue. The vast majority of women today choose to have implants placed submuscularly for a number of reasons. With submuscular placement, there is a reduced chance of capsular contracture and less interference with mammography. In addition, you're less likely to be able to feel the implants through the skin, and it may delay any future sagging. The trade-off for these benefits is a more painful recovery.

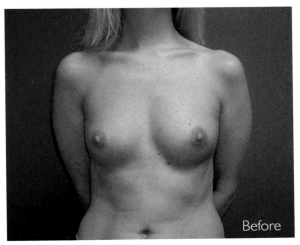

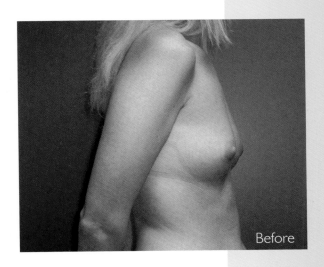

Before

Before

Age: 28. Height: 5'5"
Weight: 110. Bra size: 34 A

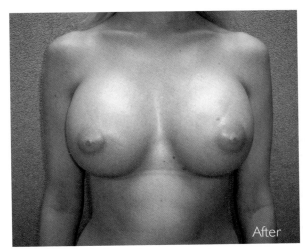

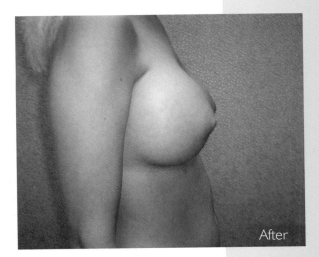

After

After

Bra size: 34 C. Six weeks postoperative
Incision: inframammary

> "Nearly every woman initially says she doesn't want her implants to be too big. However, the most common remark I hear after the surgery is, 'I wish I'd gone bigger.' For this reason, most surgeons encourage women to get implants slightly larger than what they think they want."
>
> —Steven P. Seidel, M.D.

Subglandular

When implants are placed above the muscle and beneath the breast tissue, it's called subglandular. Recovery is less painful with subglandular placement. However, you're more likely to be able to feel the implant beneath your skin, and your breasts may appear less natural than with the submuscular method. You may also be more at risk for capsular contracture. Your surgeon may suggest this method if you have a small amount of sagging and are a borderline candidate for a breast lift. When this is the case, a surgeon can place the implants lower on your chest so they're directly behind the nipple area. This way, a breast lift can be delayed.

Getting the Right Size

Getting the right-size implant requires careful planning. Implants are measured in cubic centimeters (cc) and range in size from about 125 cc to 700 cc. With some implants, the volume can't be changed once inserted; others allow for slight adjustments to increase or decrease size following surgery. There is no average or most popular size used since every woman's body and goals are unique. However, cosmetic surgeons have noticed a trend in the past decade toward larger implants.

Is Bra Size a Good Gauge?

You may think the easiest way to explain what size you want your breasts to be is to use a bra size, but bra size isn't a good gauge. No surgeon can guarantee what your bra size will be following surgery. In part, that's because every bra fits differently, and you may wear a 34C in one brand but a 36B in another. Surgeons also note that women have surprisingly different notions of what size their breasts truly are. Two women with virtually the same-size breasts may not agree on their bra size—one may claim she's an A cup while the other swears she's a C cup. This makes it very difficult for a surgeon to make a determination based on bra size alone.

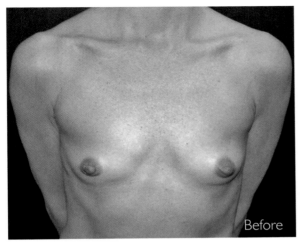

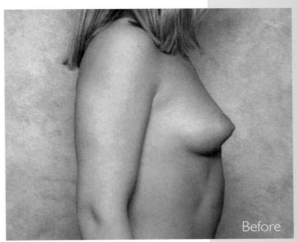

Age: 32. Height: 5' 3"
Weight: 112. Bra size: 32 A

Age: 36. Height: 5' 6"
Weight: 118. Bra size: 34 B

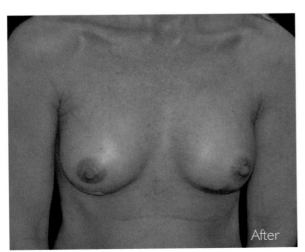

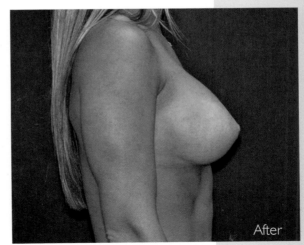

Bra size: 34 C. Eight days postoperative
Incision: inframammary. Note Steri-strips still in
place under breasts.

Bra size: 34 C. Three years postoperative
Incision: inframammary

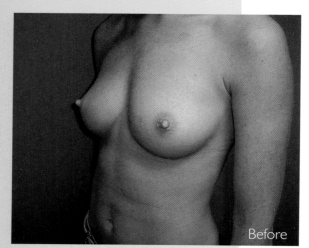

Before

Age: 18. Height: 5' 5"
Weight: 118. Bra size: 34 B

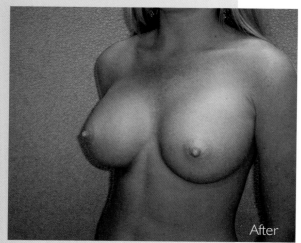

After

Bra size: 34 C. Six weeks postoperative
Incision: transaxillary

Sizing Up Your Friends' Implants

Asking friends who have breast implants what size they are may not be the best way to determine what size will work best for you. You may love the way your friend's breasts look with 350-cc implants, but that doesn't mean that 350-cc implants will look the same on you. Because every woman starts with a different frame and different amounts of breast tissue, you can't expect a particular size implant to produce the same effects on any two women.

Measuring Your Breasts

To help determine the best size implant for your body, your surgeon may take measurements of your breasts, including their diameter, the cleavage distance, the amount of breast skin, and the distance from the inframammary fold to the nipple. These measurements can help the surgeon zero in on a size that will work for you and will also reveal if your goals can be achieved. For instance, if you want to have extremely large breasts, but you have a very small frame and very little breast tissue, you may not be able to achieve the look you want. Why not? You may not have enough existing skin and tissue to cover a large implant. If, on the other hand, you have a larger frame and more existing breast tissue, a larger size may be advised. Taking your measurements into account, your doctor will discuss the options that will work best for you.

Trying on Implants

Your surgeon may suggest trying on implants in your bra to get an idea of how your breasts might look following your procedure. It may be necessary to purchase a larger bra to accommodate the test implants. Although this method is not an exact science, it can provide an indication of the implant size that will work best for you.

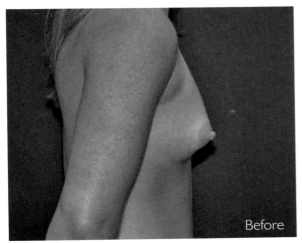

Before

Age: 28. Height: 5' 3"
Weight: 115. Bra size: 34 A

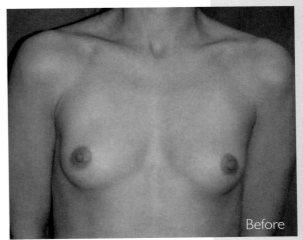

Before

Age: 34. Height: 5' 4"
Weight: 115. Bra size: 32 A

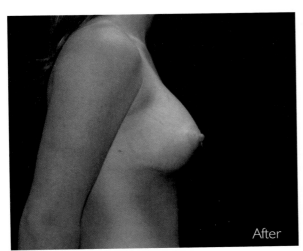

After

Bra size: 34 C. Six weeks postoperative
Incision: inframammary

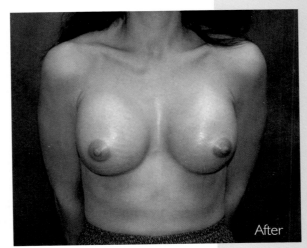

After

Bra size: 34 C. Six weeks postoperative
Incision: inframammary

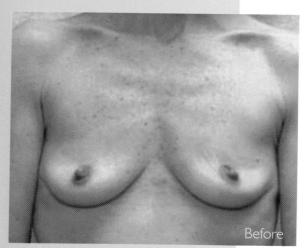

Age: 42. Height: 5' 5"
Weight: 105. Bra size: 34 A

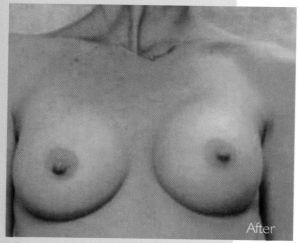

Bra size: 34 C. Five years postoperative
Incision: inframammary

Take Photos

Another way you can express what you want is to bring in photos of women from magazines or pictures of friends who have breasts similar to the size you desire. Realize that a surgeon will not be able to make your breasts look exactly like what you see in the photo. What these pictures can do is give the surgeon a better idea of what you hope to achieve.

Do Implants Interfere with Mammograms?

With traditional mammography, it is possible for implants to obscure some of the breast tissue. However, a seven-year study involving more than 1 million women revealed that yearly mammograms are effective in detecting breast cancer, whether or not a woman has implants.

To improve the detection of cancer in breasts with implants, a special mammography method called the Eklund technique has been developed.

With this technique, the mammogram technician will take a series of additional views of the breasts with the implant pushed back and the breast tissue pulled forward. This method is offered in every accredited mammography facility in the United States. If you undergo breast augmentation, it's imperative to inform the person making your mammogram appointment and the technician that you have implants. By doing so, you'll be assured that the technician will use the Eklund technique.

You should also be aware that because the breasts are squeezed during mammography, it is possible, although rare, that an implant could rupture. In spite of this rare possibility, cosmetic surgeons stress that breast augmentation patients receive yearly mammograms after the age of forty or as directed by their gynecologist or family doctor. In some instances, your surgeon may encourage you to obtain a mammogram prior to breast augmentation surgery and again approximately six months to one year after surgery to establish a baseline.

To ensure breast health, you will also be urged to perform monthly breast self-exams to look for lumps and any other changes. Your surgeon can show you how to distinguish your breast tissue from the implant.

How Long Do Implants Last?

It's impossible for any surgeon to know exactly how long your implants will last. In large part, this depends on lifestyle factors following breast augmentation—pregnancy, aging, and weight fluctuations can all affect your bustline. As for the implants themselves, there are no specific limits on the number of years you can expect them to last. However, they do not last a lifetime, and it is likely that you will need to have the implants removed or replaced at some point. In light of this, the major implant manufacturers offer lifetime product-replacement warranty policies.

Questions to Ask Your Surgeon

- What kind of implant do you recommend for me and why?

- Which incision site do you recommend and why?

- Do you recommend my implants be placed above or below the pectoral muscle?

- How do you determine the right-size implant for me?

- What is your rate of reoperation?

- What is the most common reason for reoperation?

- Will I require additional surgeries in my lifetime?

- How will my breasts look if I decide to have the implants removed?

- Will I be able to breast-feed?

- How will my breast implants look after pregnancy or breast-feeding?

- May I see before-and-after photos of patients with breasts similar to mine?

CHAPTER FIVE

Combining Breast Augmentation
with Breast Lift

5

Combining Breast Augmentation with Breast Lift

*I*f you're considering breast augmentation to enhance the appearance of your breasts, you may discover that augmentation alone won't produce the results you're hoping to achieve. Why not? If you have droopy or saggy breasts, called ptosis (pronounced: toe-sis), breast augmentation alone can't always correct this common problem. A breast lift, or mastopexy, is commonly recommended in addition to augmentation to create a more youthful contour as well as enhanced size. If you would like your breasts to look more firm as well as more full, you may want to consider this combined procedure.

What Is a Breast Lift?

A breast lift, called a mastopexy, is a surgical procedure that elevates your breasts to a higher position on your chest. The procedure restores the volume of the upper breast, tightens stretched skin, lifts sagging breast tissue, and raises droopy nipples to the center of the breast mound. The size of your areola can also be reduced with this procedure if you so desire.

If you're having a breast lift, you may also wish to have your breast size enlarged with the insertion of implants. When an augmentation is performed in conjunction with a breast lift, the procedure is known as an augmentation mastopexy.

Are You a Candidate for a Breast Lift?

If you have saggy breasts, you may be a candidate for a lift. Only your surgeon can give you a definitive answer. Plastic surgeons generally classify ptosis into three degrees, also called grades or types, and a fourth type called pseudoptosis. The degree of ptosis is determined according to the position of the nipple in comparison with the inframammary fold, the crease below the breast. In a normal breast with no ptosis, the nipple lies above the inframammary fold and on the mound of the breast.

Degrees of Ptosis

First degree (Grade 1): minimal or mild droop; the nipple is level with the inframammary fold.

Second degree (Grade 2): moderate droop; the nipple falls below the inframammary fold but is still above the lowest part of the breast.

Third degree (Grade 3): major, advanced, or severe droop; the nipple falls below the inframammary fold, is below the lowest part of the breast, and points downward.

Pseudoptosis: the nipple is above the inframammary fold, but the breast tissue falls below it.

A breast lift can provide remarkable results for women of all ages, provided you're healthy and you have a good attitude and realistic expectations. If you're like the majority of patients who can benefit from this procedure, you're probably in your thirties or forties and have lost volume and firmness due to pregnancy and breast-feeding. If you're over fifty, you might consider the procedure to reverse the effects of aging as well as childbirth. If you're a younger

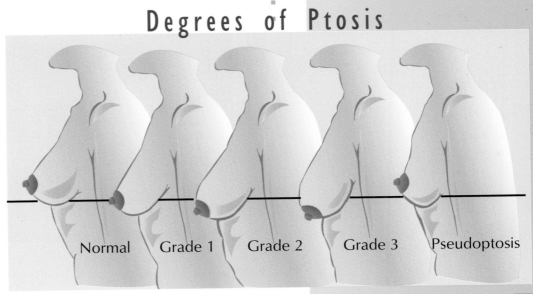

Degrees of Ptosis

Normal   Grade 1   Grade 2   Grade 3   Pseudoptosis

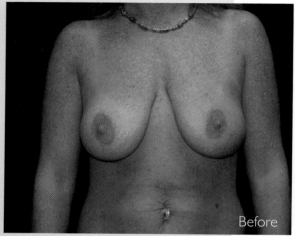

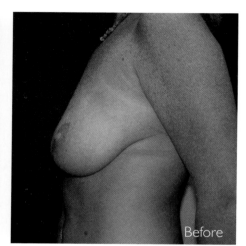

Age: 38. Height: 5' 4"
Weight: 141. Bra size: 36 B

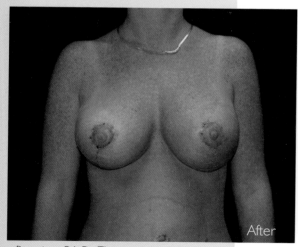

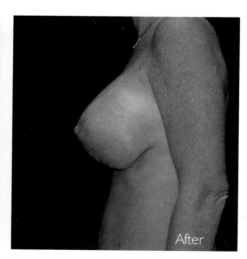

Bra size: 36 D. Three weeks postoperative
Procedure: vertical breast lift with augmentation

woman who has had unwanted sagging since puberty, you might seek out a lift to correct this inherited trait.

When a Breast Lift May Not Be for You

In some instances, a breast lift may not be appropriate for you. If you're planning to become pregnant in the future, most doctors would advise postponing surgery until after you're finished bearing children. This advice is based on the fact that pregnancy can cause breasts that have been lifted to sag again. If you're overweight, and planning to lose weight in the near future, it may be better to delay surgery until after you've stabilized your weight. Weight loss can diminish breast volume and produce loose skin and sagging tissue, which is exactly what is being corrected with a breast lift.

If the idea of having permanent scars on your

breasts is unacceptable to you, a breast lift may not be for you. It's important for anyone considering an augmentation/lift procedure to understand that the resulting scars are larger and more visible than those associated with breast augmentation alone. In general, the more sagging you have, the more scarring you can expect. Fortunately, the scars associated with a breast lift are located in areas where they are easily concealed by a bra. Even so, considering that you're seeking cosmetic surgery to make your breasts more attractive, permanent scars may not fit into your ideal vision. Ultimately, you're the only one who can decide how much scarring you're willing to live with as a trade-off for firmer breasts.

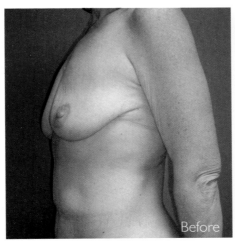
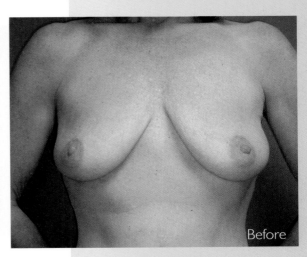

Age: 43. Height: 5' 4"
Weight: 141. Bra size: 34 C

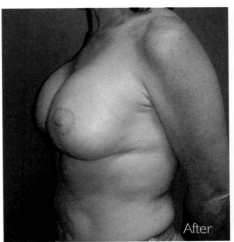
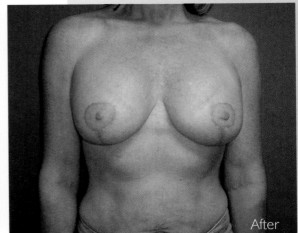

Bra size: 34 D. Two months postoperative
Procedure: Vertical breast lift with
augmentation

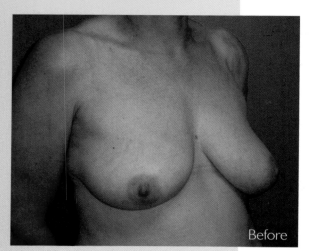

Age: 52. Height: 5' 2"
Weight: 134. Bra size: 36 D

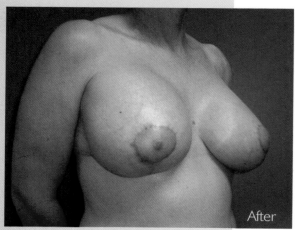

Bra size: 36 DD
Procedure: vertical breast lift with augmentation
Two months postoperative

Your Breast Augmentation with Breast Lift Procedure

When these two procedures are combined, surgery takes about two to three hours. After you're adequately anesthetized, the surgeon makes an incision on the breast. The most common incision sites are: around the areola; from the areola straight down to the inframammary fold; across the crease of the inframammary fold—or some combination of these three. The surgeon then removes a conservative amount of excess skin from the breast.

Using the same incision, he or she will create a pocket for the implant and insert it into the breast. With the implant in place, the nipple/areola complex and the breast tissue connected to it are raised from a droopy location to a more natural position on the breast mound. In some instances, the size of the areola is reduced as well. Any additional excess skin is removed, and the remaining skin is redraped around the breast tissue and the implant. The incision is then closed with sutures.

Breast Lift Techniques

When augmentation is performed at the same time as a breast lift, your surgeon will choose from several breast lift techniques. Each case is highly individual and the technique chosen will depend on a combination of the degree of ptosis and the implant size. In general, the higher the degree of ptosis, the more invasive the technique will be. Conversely, the larger the implant, the less invasive the technique will be. In each of the following techniques, a breast implant can be inserted through the breast lift incision.

Vertical

The vertical technique is also called the "lollipop" technique due to the shape of the scar it leaves. This approach works better for women with mild to moderate sagging in which the nipple is near the inframammary fold. When using this technique, the surgeon makes two incisions—one around the border of the areola and one vertically from the bottom edge of the areola down to near the inframammary fold. Excess skin is removed, and the areola/nipple complex and attached breast tissue are raised. The breast tissue is sutured to the chest wall for additional support and the remaining skin is stitched together, resulting in a lollipop-shaped scar.

Wise Pattern

The Wise pattern incision is most commonly-used when the degree of sagging is severe and requires considerable skin removal and elevation of the nipple. This procedure has the ability to correct the greatest degree of sag by using both vertical and horizontal skin excisions below the nipple. This technique involves an incision around the periphery of the areola, a vertical incision, and a horizontal incision that follows the inframammary fold. The horizontal incision can be continued along the side to remove excess tissue that extends either towards the back or the underarm. The approach is also often referred to as the "inverted T" technique or "anchor" technique because of the shape of the scar it leaves on the breasts.

Periareolar

The periareolar technique is best suited for women who have smaller breasts and only a moderate degree of droop. With this technique, the surgeon makes a circular or oval incision around the entire edge of the areola and another larger one slightly beyond the areola. The skin between the two incisions is

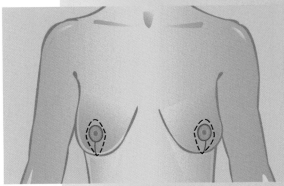

Vertical (Lollipop) Incision

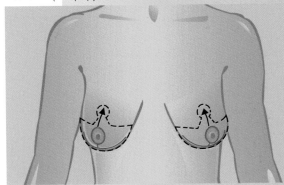

Wise Pattern (Anchor) Incision

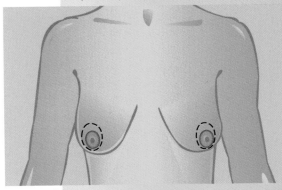

Periareolar Incision

removed—the excised portion of skin resembles the shape of a doughnut. The nipple/areola complex and breast tissue attached to it are lifted to a more natural position. The breast tissue is sutured to the chest wall to give it more support, and the remaining skin is pulled together around the areola. The surgeon closes the incision by stitching around the areola and pulling those stitches together as if tightening a purse string.

You may hear the periareolar technique referred to by other names such as "doughnut" mastopexy, "concentric" mastopexy, or "draw-string" mastopexy.

Crescent

The crescent technique involves making an incision along the borderline of the upper portion of the areola and removing excess skin from the upper portion of the breast. The nipple/areola complex is raised to a new, more pleasing position on the breast. This lift is seldom used since it limits the amount of lift you can attain with it.

Breast Lift with Implants Procedure

With each breast lift technique, a breast implant can be inserted through the breast lift incision. When augmentation is going to be combined with a breast lift, you and your surgeon will still need to make many of the same decisions regarding type, shape, size, and texture of implant to use and where to place it within the breast. With the combined procedure, the breast lift technique your surgeon chooses will depend on a combination of your degree of ptosis as well as the size of implant you choose.

One benefit of performing augmentation with a breast lift is that an implant will fill out some of the saggy skin. This may allow the surgeon to perform a more minor variation of a breast lift, leaving you with less scarring than if you were having a breast lift alone. For example, if you have third-degree ptosis, your surgeon would probably recommend a Wise-pattern incision. But when an implant is inserted as part of the

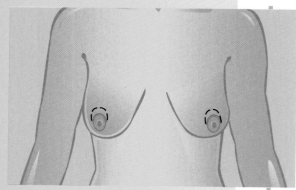

Crescent Incision

procedure, your surgeon may be able to use the vertical technique instead, freeing you from the horizontal incision along the inframammary fold.

Getting the Right Size

When combining augmentation with a lift, achieving the ideal breast size, placement, and symmetry isn't an exact science. Simply said, an augmentation/lift is a more complex procedure. With augmentation alone, a surgeon only has to position the implants and fill them to the ideal proportions. With an augmentation/lift, the surgeon must also remove breast tissue and excess skin and reposition the nipple/areola complex and connected breast tissue onto the augmented breasts. It's important to discuss this with your surgeon so you have realistic expectations about the outcome of the procedure. A surgeon may use some of the same sizing techniques discussed earlier to help you achieve the proportions you desire.

How Long Will a Breast Lift Last?

Ideally, the results from a breast lift should last for many years. However, future pregnancies and significant weight fluctuations could dramatically alter the appearance of your new breasts in unpredictable and undesirable ways. Also, aging and the effects of gravity will eventually take their toll, and unwanted sagging can return. In the same way that larger natural breasts are more likely to develop ptosis due to their weight, larger implants accelerate the recurrence of ptosis. If you already have very loose skin with little elasticity, sagging is more likely to recur. One advantage of combining a lift with breast augmentation is that implants may help delay any future sagging.

Questions to Ask Your Surgeon

- Can breast augmentation alone give me the results I want?

- Will I see better results from a combined augmentation and lift?

- Which breast lift technique do you recommend for me?

- How much scarring can I expect from the procedure?

- If I'm planning to get pregnant in the future, should I wait to have the procedure?

- Will sagging return after I have the procedure?

CHAPTER SIX

Recovering from Breast Augmentation Surgery

Recovering from Breast Augmentation Surgery

*F*ollowing your breast augmentation procedure, the recovery process begins. In the days and weeks ahead, your body will heal itself from the effects of surgery. With each passing day, you'll probably look and feel better. By taking good care of yourself during this important phase, you can help keep the healing process on track. Eventually, after a full recovery, you can begin to enjoy the new contours of your body.

Immediately after Surgery

After your breast augmentation procedure, you will remain in the recovery room for one to four hours, depending on when the anesthetic wears off and when you're fully awake. Most breast augmentation patients can go home after about an hour. Under no circumstances will you be allowed to drive after surgery, so be sure you've arranged for a driver and at-home caregiver as detailed in your preoperative instructions.

Following breast augmentation surgery, you will most likely be placed in a surgical bra and possibly a compression bandage. Depending on the incision site, you may also have gauze dressings or Steri-Strips. The bra is used to hold the implants in the proper position. If used, the compression bandage is applied to the top half of the breasts in an effort to keep the implants as low as possible during the initial healing phase. This is necessary because implants placed submuscularly typically ride high on the chest initially.

Instructions to Follow

To speed healing and make your recovery more comfortable, your doctor will give you detailed postoperative instructions. Following these instructions will speed the healing process so you can get back in the swing of things as soon as possible. Make sure your caregiver is also aware of the instructions since the effects of surgery and anesthesia may prevent you from remembering all the details.

The specific instructions you receive depend on several factors, including your incision site, whether you've had a breast lift as well as an augmentation, and your surgeon's own experience and preferences. Here are some common postoperative instructions for breast augmentation and breast lift with augmentation.

- Do not remove your surgical bra, compression bandage, or gauze dressings unless instructed to do so (the bra and compression bandage can be removed when showering; see below in list for specifics). Resist the urge to peek under the bra or wrap, and don't loosen the bandage. It is intended to be very tight. However, if the bra feels too tight, you may be instructed to change to one that feels more comfortable. A bra that's too tight can result in ulceration of the skin.

- Wear the bra day and night for at least one to two weeks as instructed, then just during the day until instructed otherwise.

- Keep any dressings, including the bra, compression bandage, and gauze dressings, as clean and dry as possible.

- If you have Steri-Strips along the incisions, do not remove them. They will come off on their own.

- Try to sleep on your back for about the first week in order to keep your implants in the proper position. However, if it's impossible for you to get any sleep on your back, sleep in any position that's comfortable for you.

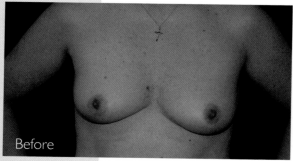

Before

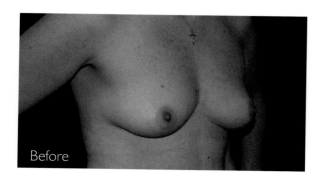

Before

Age: 48. Height: 5'4"
Weight: 136. Bra size: 34B

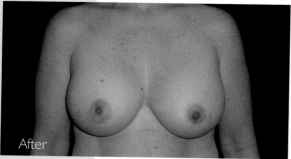

After

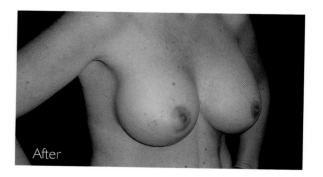

After

Bra size: 34DD. Three months postoperative
Incision: inframammary

- When you're in bed, keep your head and shoulders elevated with a couple of pillows to help eliminate swelling and pain.

- Avoid bending over, straining, or any other activities that put increased pressure on the chest for the first week to prevent unnecessary swelling and bleeding.

- You may take gentle walks within a few days, but avoid aerobic exercise for about three weeks.

- Don't lift anything heavier than a glass of water, and don't raise your arms over your head.

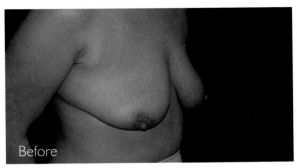

Before

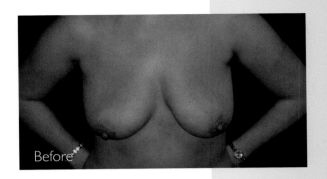

Before

Age: 40. Height: 5'6"
Weight: 140. Bra size: 34C

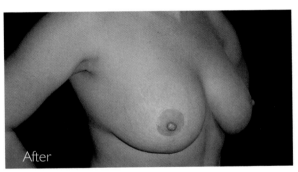

After

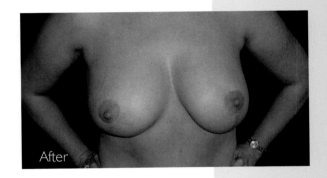

After

Bra size: 36D. One year postoperative
Procedure: vertical breast lift with augmentation

- Drink plenty of fluids. Even if you don't have much of an appetite, which is normal, your body needs fluids.

- If you feel nauseated, drink carbonated sodas and eat crackers to settle your stomach. If your stomach feels okay, start with a bland diet and progress to your normal diet.

- Don't drink any alcohol for about ten days because it can dilate the blood vessels and increase postoperative bleeding. Also avoid alcohol while taking pain medication or sedatives as this can be a dangerous combination.

- Avoid smoking and secondhand smoke for about ten days after surgery, especially if you're an augmentation/lift patient.

- Protect your breasts from impact or trauma during your recovery.

- You may shower one to two days after surgery but may be asked to refrain from letting the water hit your breasts directly. You may remove the bra and compression bandage while you shower.

- Protect your scars from the sun by wearing sunscreen. Sunlight can interfere with the proper fading of scars, which can take up to a year to fade completely.

- Avoid wearing an underwire bra for up to six months. The wires may impede healing and can be uncomfortable.

Your First Post-Op Appointment

Some surgeons will ask you to return for your first follow-up visit within the first few days after surgery. If your doctor makes this request, he or she will most likely remove the surgical bra, compression bandage, and gauze dressings to examine your breasts and incisions. At this time, he or she will determine if it's necessary for you to continue wearing the bandage if you were given one. In general, you will be asked to continue wearing the bra day and night for one to two weeks.

Follow-Up Examinations

You will usually have a follow-up visit with your surgeon approximately one to two weeks after surgery. At this visit, your surgeon will examine your breasts and incisions and may remove stitches. Based upon the examination, you will be given further instructions on wearing the bra and the bandage if you were given one.

At this time, your doctor may recommend that you begin breast massage as a way to decrease your chances of developing capsular contracture. There is some debate within the medical community about the effectiveness of breast massage in reducing incidences of capsular contracture. Whether it is effective or not, there is no harm in doing it. It's best to follow your doctor's instructions about breast massage.

In the Weeks Ahead

As the healing process continues in the weeks ahead, your life will return to normal. You can generally return to work within a few days after your procedure, but you should avoid strenuous activities that could raise your pulse or blood pressure for at least two to three weeks. If you're an augmentation/lift patient, your recovery will require more time than that of an augmentation-only patient. Ask your doctor for a specific timetable for resuming normal activities, such as:

- Driving a car

- Returning to office work

- Resuming light housework

- Resuming nonstrenuous activities

- Resuming sexual activity

- Resuming strenuous physical activities and housework

- Going swimming

Remember that every woman is different, and you may recover faster or slower than the timetable indicates. Your best bet is to avoid activities that cause pain. To keep your recovery on track, follow your doctor's instructions meticulously. By doing so, you'll be back to normal and enjoying your new physique sooner.

Possible Side Effects of Breast Augmentation

As your body heals during your recovery, you may experience some common side effects associated with breast augmentation. These side effects are usually temporary in nature. Following breast augmentation, each breast heals differently. Certain side effects may affect only one of your breasts, or both of them but at different levels of intensity. This is normal.

- *Chest pain*: You can expect to feel pain throughout the chest area following breast augmentation, especially if your implants have been placed submuscularly. Sometimes, the pain radiates down into the arms or back. The medication your doctor has prescribed should alleviate the pain to allow you a more restful recovery. If the medication doesn't ease your pain, contact your doctor.

- *Shooting or burning pains*: You may experience temporary shooting or burning pains at the sides of your breasts. This is associated with the healing and regeneration of sensory nerves.

- *Asymmetry*: Because each breast heals differently, your breasts may not look exactly alike initially. One of your breasts may appear larger than the other due to more swelling, or the shapes may differ slightly. These differences are usually resolved once you've healed completely.

- *Swelling*: Your breasts will probably feel swollen and heavy for at least several weeks following surgery. Realize that it may be six months or longer until your breasts assume their final shape and size.

- *Tightness*: As your skin adjusts to your new breast size, you may feel a sense of tightness throughout the chest area.

- *Numbness*: One or both of your nipples or other areas of your breasts may feel numb temporarily.

- *Hypersensitive nipples*: One or both of your nipples may temporarily be extremely sensitive to touch.

- *High breast shape*: Implants placed submuscularly may ride high on the chest for some time before settling into a more natural position. Wearing the compression bandage as directed will help implants achieve proper placement.

- *Bruising*: You may find some bruising on one or both of your breasts, but this usually fades quickly.

- *Sloshing*: You may feel or hear "sloshing" within your breast after augmentation. Don't worry. It isn't the saline in your implant sloshing around. This harmless side effect is a result of natural fluids accumulating around your implant. These fluids are normally absorbed by the body within a matter of weeks.

- *Shiny skin*: The swelling after surgery may cause the skin of your breasts to look shiny. Your skin will return to normal as the swelling subsides.

Risks and Potential Complications of Breast Augmentation

Capsular Contracture

Capsular contracture is the most common complication associated with breast augmentation. When any foreign object, such as a breast implant, is placed in the body, scar tissue forms around it as a natural part of the healing process. In most women, this scar tissue doesn't cause any problems. However, in some instances, this scar tissue contracts and squeezes the implant.

This contraction results in varying degrees of undesirable firmness and can lead to pain or distortion of the breast shape. Most cases of this condition are mild and don't require intervention. In the rarer severe cases, it can require additional surgery to remove the scarring or to remove and possibly replace the implant. According to one study assessing complication rates for breast augmentation patients, 11 percent of patients experienced some degree of capsular contracture within five years of their augmentation procedure.

Capsular contracture can occur at any time following breast augmentation surgery and may affect only one breast or both of them. At this time, plastic surgeons don't know the exact causes of capsular contracture and are continuing to investigate. However, surgeons do know that implants placed submuscularly are less likely to develop the condition than implants placed subglandularly. However, when textured implants are used in the submuscular position, the frequency of capsular contracture is about the same as with subglandular placement.

Rupture/Deflation

Over time, an implant may rupture, leak, or deflate. One study shows that 10 percent of patients experienced implant deflation within the first seven years following augmentation surgery. If a saline-filled implant ruptures, it will leak and deflate either immediately or over a couple days. Deflation of a saline implant isn't harmful because the body simply absorbs the saline. You can tell that the implant has deflated because your breast will lose its shape and size.

If a silicone-gel implant ruptures and leaks, you may not be able to notice it. The silicone gel will remain in or near the implant despite the rupture. If you or your surgeon have reason to believe a silicone-gel implant has ruptured, an MRI is considered the best technique to make such a determination. Causes of deflation include capsular contracture, normal wear and tear, trauma to the breast, compression during mammography, and, rarely, damage to the implant during surgery. If an implant ruptures or deflates, it can only be replaced with additional surgery.

Disappointment with Size

Despite your surgeon's best efforts to provide you with the size you desire, you may decide after surgery that you would prefer your breasts to be larger or smaller. Surgeons say that most women who decide to change their size after surgery choose a bigger size. Some implants are designed to allow a surgeon to add or remove saline in a simple office procedure for up to six months following surgery. With other types of implants, a second surgery will be necessary to alter the size.

Implant Visibility/Palpability

In some instances, you may be able to see the edges of your implant or feel it through the skin. This is more common with subglandular placement, and also with large implants that are placed in someone with a very small frame and little natural breast tissue.

Wrinkling

The free-flowing liquid saline within an implant can create waves that appear like wrinkles or ripples through the skin. Thin women with little original breast tissue and those with textured implants are more likely to experience wrinkling.

Asymmetry

No two breasts are exactly alike before surgery, and no two breasts are exactly alike after augmentation surgery. Minor differences are usually acceptable. If the difference in size, shape, or nipple position following surgery is major, you may want to consider a surgical revision.

Implant Malposition

Sometimes, an implant isn't placed in the best position, or it shifts or rotates out of its ideal location. With round implants, rotating may not be noticeable, but with anatomical implants, rotating can create breasts with undesirable shapes. Minor shifts may be acceptable, but major shifts may require a second procedure to reposition the implant.

Altered Nipple/Breast Sensation

Following surgery, the feeling in your nipples or breasts can be heightened or reduced. Changes in sensation may be caused by surgeons cutting through very tiny nerves while making incisions or by implants placing pressure on nerves within the breast. When sensitivity is lost, it is regained within a year or two in about 85 percent of cases.

Capsule Calcification

The capsule that forms around the implant may develop calcium deposits. This usually occurs several years after an augmentation procedure. The calcium deposits can show up on mammograms and be mistaken for cancer, possibly requiring a biopsy or surgical procedure to rule out cancer. The calcium deposits can also obscure the visibility of other, possibly cancerous lesions in traditional mammography. As mentioned in chapter 4, a special mammography method, called the Eklund technique, can help view this breast tissue.

Interference with Breast-Feeding

As mentioned earlier, the periareolar incision may reduce the ability to breast-feed successfully. The other types of incisions, transaxillary, inframammary, and transumbilical, should have little effect on the ability to breast-feed.

Silicone in Breast Milk

It is unknown at this time whether or not silicone from the breast-implant shell can be transmitted to the breast milk.

Interference with Mammography

As mentioned, it is possible for breast implants to interfere with traditional mammography. However, the special viewing method already discussed in chapter 4, the Eklund technique, has improved the ability to detect breast cancer in women with implants. A major study involving more than 1 million women showed that mammography is effective in detecting breast cancer in women with breast implants. Other studies have shown that when breast cancer is detected in women with implants, it is at the same stage as cancers found in women without implants.

Breast Cancer

There is no hard evidence connecting breast implants with breast cancer. Studies show that the rate of breast cancer among women with implants is the same or even slightly less than among women without implants.

Connective-Tissue Disorders

Numerous studies indicate that silicone-gel implants do not cause or contribute to connective-tissue disorders, such as rheumatoid arthritis, fibromyalgia, or lupus. Likewise, saline-filled implants are not linked with these diseases.

Chronic Pain

In rare cases, breast pain does not subside and becomes chronic. If your pain is severe or doesn't go away following the recovery period, contact your doctor.

Exposure/Extrusion of Implant

This very rare complication occurs when there is erosion of an implant through the skin or a scar. Causes may include having thin skin or having an insufficient amount of breast tissue to adequately cover the implant. Capsular contracture, infection, and severe rippling may also be contributing factors.

Synmastia

In very rare cases, the skin between the two breasts pulls away from the breastbone, reducing or eliminating the appearance of cleavage. If this unusual complication develops, it may require additional surgery.

Tissue Necrosis

As mentioned earlier, tissue necrosis, or skin death, may occur when an area of skin loses its blood supply. This type of complication usually occurs at the site of the incision, and occurs more often with larger incisions. Since breast lifts involve larger incisions, you're more at risk if you're having a breast lift with augmentation rather than an augmentation alone. Because smoking compromises skin circulation, smokers are also more at risk. Tissue that is painful and blue, purple, or gray may mark the early stages of tissue death.

Incision Complications

Incisions that separate are not very common with augmentation, but are much more likely with augmentation/lift. These wounds usually heal

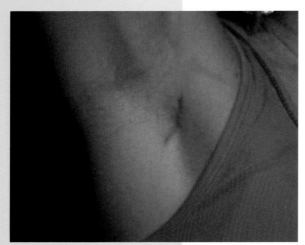

Scar from transaxillary (armpit) incision for breast implant six weeks after surgery. The scar maturation process takes 6 to 12 months.

with minor treatment by the surgeon and don't require additional surgery, but they may prolong the healing process.

Infection

Thanks to the antibiotics used in the operating room and during recovery, infections are very rare, affecting only about 1 percent of breast augmentation patients. Redness, extreme pain, and significant swelling in the breast are symptoms of an infection. If an infection doesn't respond to antibiotics, the implant may have to be temporarily removed in an additional surgery. The implant is generally replaced in a follow-up surgery in approximately six months.

Toxic Shock Syndrome

In extremely rare cases, toxic shock syndrome has been reported in breast augmentation patients. This life-threatening condition's symptoms include rash, fainting, diarrhea, vomiting, and sudden fever. If you experience any of these symptoms, notify your doctor immediately.

Postoperative Bleeding

A little bruising from postoperative bleeding is normal, but if unusual bleeding occurs, the breast will suddenly become painful and swell to a size much larger than the other breast. Contact your doctor immediately as this rare occurrence usually requires additional surgery to stop the bleeding.

Hematoma/Seroma

If a hematoma or seroma develops in the breast, it can cause swelling, pain, and bruising, and may contribute to capsular contracture and infection. The body can usually absorb small hematomas and seromas on its own, but large ones may need to be drained through the use of drainage tubes or with an additional surgical procedure. An implant can be damaged during the draining process, resulting in rupture and possibly deflation.

Follow-Up Care

As you return to normal over the following days, weeks, and months, your breasts will require less and less follow-up care. Eventually, unless you develop a complication, they won't need much follow-up care at all, and you'll probably stop thinking about them on a day-to-day basis.

In the first weeks and months following your surgery, you will probably have several follow-up visits with your surgeon to remove stitches and monitor your recovery. After the initial recovery phase, your follow-up visits will become more infrequent. Even if you are feeling fine and don't have any problems with your implants, it's important to keep these appointments. Your surgeon can detect potential complications and take action to correct them before they become problematic.

Implant Removal

At some point during your lifetime, you will likely undergo additional surgery to remove and possibly replace your implants. The top reasons for implant removal are patient choice (42 percent), implant deflation (32 percent), and capsular contracture (9 percent). This is according to the Post Approval Survey Study (PASS), a clinical study sponsored by Inamed, a breast-implant manufacturer, which tracked women for seven years following breast augmentation surgery.

The vast majority of women who undergo implant removal get replacement implants. In fact, implant removal with replacement is the most common additional surgical procedure for breast augmentation patients (34 percent), according to Inamed's A95 study, which assessed complication rates for five years following breast augmentation. The same study shows that only 2 percent of additional surgical procedures involved implant removal without replacement.

CHAPTER SEVEN

Liposuction

7

Liposuction

*D*o you have bulges or pockets of fat that just won't go away? Have you tried dieting and exercise but can't get rid of this stubborn fat? If so, you may want to consider liposuction. Liposuction has emerged in recent years as the single most popular cosmetic surgical procedure performed in the United States. Each year, nearly half a million people have liposuction to remove unwanted fat and redefine body proportions.

What makes liposuction so popular? The procedure can produce dramatic changes in your body contour, often improving what years of diet and exercise couldn't achieve. Inconspicuous scars and a relatively short recovery period add to its appeal. With these advantages, it's easy to see why millions of Americans, and perhaps you, are considering liposuction as a way to achieve a more sleek, streamlined appearance.

Commonly Treated Areas of the Body

Body contouring with liposuction can be performed on several areas of the body, but the most commonly treated sites include the abdomen, thighs, hips, and buttocks. Other parts of the body can also show marked improvement following the procedure. If you're like most women, you may wish to have more than one area treated at the same time.

Abdomen

Liposuction of the abdomen can create a flatter stomach. Suctioning of the abdomen may be restricted to the area below the belly button or may include the upper abdomen if necessary. As a rule, a surgeon can suction only the fat you can "pinch" on your belly.

Thighs

Liposuction of the thighs is performed to make the legs look more attractive. Most surgeons treat the thighs as two separate areas: inner thighs and outer thighs. Treatment of the inner or outer thighs often includes suctioning of excess fat on the back of the thighs and buttocks as well. In general, treatment of the outer thighs tends to produce more even results than liposuction of the inner thighs. Why? The thin, delicate skin on the inner thighs is more likely to reveal any irregularities or unevenness under the skin.

Hips

Liposuction of the hips can enhance your silhouette. Suctioning of fat from the hips is often combined with fat removal from the thighs or buttocks.

Buttocks

Liposuction of the buttocks can improve its size and shape. Because the rear end serves as a cushion while sitting on hard surfaces, surgeons are often conservative in the volume of fat they'll remove in this area.

Other Areas

The part of your body your surgeon may refer to as *flanks* are areas often treated successfully with liposuction. A flank refers to the fleshy part on the side of your body between ribs and hip. Other areas which can be contoured with liposuction include the inner knees, calves, ankles, upper arms, and back. In the early days of liposuction, fat removal in these areas often

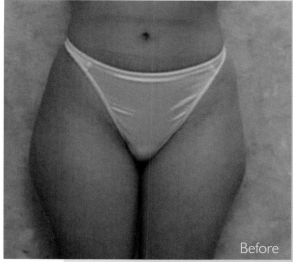

Before

Age: 35

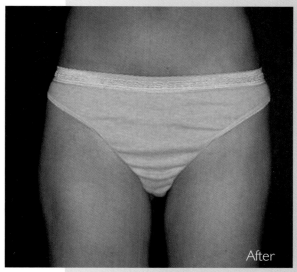

After

Procedure: Liposuction to the hips and outer thighs

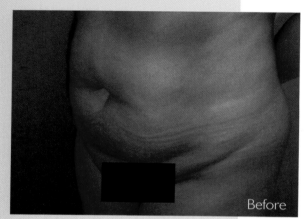

Age: 31

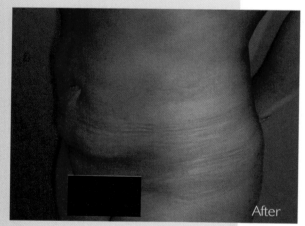

Procedure: Liposuction to abdomen and flanks, area between ribs and hips.

produced unsatisfactory results. Thanks to improvements in surgical techniques during the past years, these areas routinely produce good results.

Removing Fat with Liposuction

Within the body, there are three kinds of fat: superficial, subcutaneous, and intra-abdominal. Although all three of these types of body fat *can* be removed with liposuction, it is not advised for removal of intra-abdominal fat. Superficial fat is a thin layer of fat found directly below the skin. This layer of fat contributes to the dimpling and puckering called cellulite that is often found on the thighs and buttocks. Subcutaneous fat is a thick layer of fat found deeper in the body. It's this deep, thick layer of fat that's responsible for producing visible bulges on the tummy, hips, and thighs. Subcutaneous fat generally contributes to a "pear-shaped" body that's common among women. Intra-abdominal fat is interspersed throughout the internal organs of the abdomen, often producing an "apple-shaped" body that is more common among men.

Liposuction is primarily aimed at removing the thick, subcutaneous layer of fat. When targeting this layer of fat, liposuction produces its best results. When the procedure is performed on the thin, superficial layer of fat, irregularities are more likely to be seen. However, advances in surgical techniques and instruments have vastly improved the results.

Are You a Candidate for Liposuction?

Anyone who has localized fat deposits that don't respond to diet and exercise may benefit from liposuction. The best candidates are at or near their ideal weight, but even if you're moderately overweight, you may still see improvements with liposuction.

To determine whether liposuction is right for you, your surgeon will consider the volume and location of fat on your body. In addition, the quality of your skin tone will come into play. Because the skin must contract to adapt to the new contour following liposuction, having adequate skin elasticity is necessary for the best results. In general, younger people tend to have better skin tone with more elasticity. However, this doesn't rule out the procedure if you're approaching middle age or beyond. In fact, millions of Americans of all ages have experienced remarkable improvements from liposuction. Regardless of your age, your surgeon will determine if your skin has enough elasticity to achieve your goals.

When Liposuction May Not Be for You

Sometimes, liposuction may need to be combined with other procedures to produce the results you desire. And in some instances, liposuction might not be the right procedure for you. If any of the following are among your reasons for having liposuction, you may want to rethink having this procedure.

- **You are obese or you want to lose weight**. Liposuction is not a treatment for obesity nor is it a solution for weight loss. Limits on the amount of fat that can safely be removed prevent plastic surgeons from treating the obese. In addition, the procedure isn't designed to remove fat that is evenly distributed on an overweight body. If you are obese or overweight, doctors will likely recommend you try diet and exercise to lose weight, or in some cases, may suggest a surgical procedure, such as gastric bypass.

- **You have loose skin**. If your skin lacks elasticity, liposuction alone may not achieve your goals. After fat removal, loose skin may appear even more droopy and saggy. In most cases, if you're troubled by loose skin and localized fat deposits, your surgeon may suggest a tummy tuck, thigh lift, or lower-body lift that will remove excess skin in addition to excess fat.

- **Your goal is to remove stretch marks**. Liposuction can't remove or reduce the appearance of stretch marks. Your surgeon may suggest a tummy tuck to remove stretch marks.

- **You're looking for a solution for cellulite**. Liposuction will not improve the appearance of cellulite (the common, unattractive "cottage cheese" appearance of the skin on the hips, thighs, and buttocks).

- **You have scarring from a previous surgery**. Liposuction may not be recommended if scarring exists in the area to be treated. Scar tissue may interfere with fat removal in that specific area and leave you with less-than-optimal results.

If you've recently gained or lost weight, your surgeon may recommend that you stabilize your weight for six to twelve months before undergoing the procedure.

Your Liposuction Procedure

The liposuction procedure routinely takes about forty-five minutes to two hours. However, depending on the amount of fat to be removed and the technique used, it could take onger. After you are fully sedated, your surgeon will make several small incisions in the areas where fat will be removed. Using one of several surgical techniques, your surgeon will prepare the fat cells for removal.

Following this step, a suction tube is inserted through the incisions, and excess fat is literally vacuumed out along with small amounts of blood and body fluids. Avoiding any contact with neighboring organs, nerves, blood vessels, or connective tissue, your surgeon will continue moving the suction tube throughout the fat until the appropriate amount has been removed.

Once the ideal contour is achieved, your surgeon may or may not close the incisions with nonabsorbable sutures that will need to be removed in the doctor's office. Surgeons who choose to use sutures claim that it decreases the amount of drainage, which can be profuse and messy. Those who prefer not to close the tiny incisions with sutures claim that the additional drainage reduces swelling.

Incisions

The incisions made in liposuction are very small, usually measuring only one-eighth to one-half inch each. The number of incisions you will require depends on the number of areas to be treated and the amount of fat to be removed. Whenever possible, incisions are hidden in the pubic hair or in convenient folds or skin creases, such as under the fold of the buttocks or in the belly button. When incisions can't be hidden, the resulting scars are usually inconspicuous.

Volume of Fat Removed

To determine the volume of fat to be removed, a surgeon will look at your body size, your age, and your overall health. As a general rule, it's considered safe to limit the amount of fat to be removed in a single operation to about five liters, which is about eleven pounds.

With advances in surgical techniques, a growing number of surgeons have started performing large-volume fat removal of more than five liters in a single operation. Large-volume fat removal carries greater risks, including increased blood loss, longer operating times, higher doses of anesthetics, and greater stress to the body. Because of increased blood loss, large-volume fat removal could require the need for a blood transfusion. If you will be having more than five liters of fat removed, you may be encouraged to donate your own blood prior to surgery in case you need a transfusion. As a safer approach, your surgeon may suggest an additional liposuction procedure in about six months to remove fat in excess of five liters.

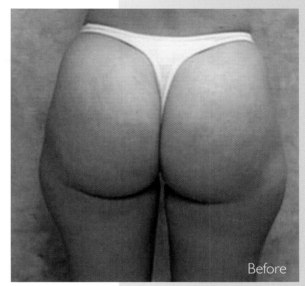

Before

Age: 28

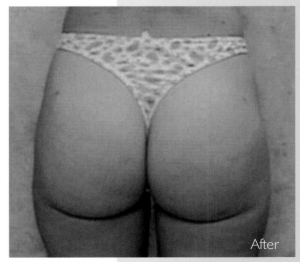

After

Procedure: Liposuction to buttocks, thighs, and hips

> "One of the most beneficial things you can do after liposuction is lose weight in the immediate postoperative period. Why? The fat cells that remain can be shrunk, enhancing the new contours."
>
> —C. Andrew Salzberg, M.D.

Liposuction Techniques

Tumescent

The most common technique used for the procedure today is tumescent liposuction. With this technique, surgeons prepare the fat cells for removal by injecting various quantities of fluid through the incisions into the areas to be treated. The fluid generally contains a mix of saline, epinephrine (a drug that contracts blood vessels), and lidocaine (a local anesthetic). The effects of the fluid facilitate fat removal, reduce blood loss, and improve the final results.

The term tumescent means swollen and accurately describes the appearance of the area to be treated immediately following injection of the fluid. Considering that the volume of fluid injected may be as much as three times the volume of fat to be removed, it's easy to understand why the treated area would appear swollen. Depending on the volume of fluid injected, this technique may also be called wet or superwet.

Ultrasound-Assisted Liposuction (UAL)

In some instances, surgeons may opt to use ultrasound in conjunction with the tumescent technique. With this technique, an ultrasonic probe is inserted into the fat layer through the incisions. Ultrasonic vibrations from the probe create heat and cause the fat cells to emulsify or melt, facilitating their removal. This technique allows larger amounts of fat to be removed with less blood loss. For this reason, surgeons often choose this technique when performing large-volume liposuction. UAL also facilitates the removal of fat in areas where tissues are more fibrous and normally harder to treat, such as the upper abdomen and back.

Other variations of UAL include external ultrasound and VASER-assisted liposuction. External ultrasound transmits ultrasound waves through the skin using a special emitter to liquefy the fat cells. VASER-assisted liposuction is a system which uses ultrasound energy to break up and emulsify fat, leaving intact surrounding tissue such as nerves, blood vessels and connective tissue.

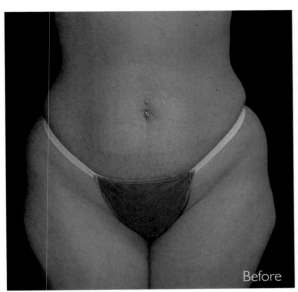
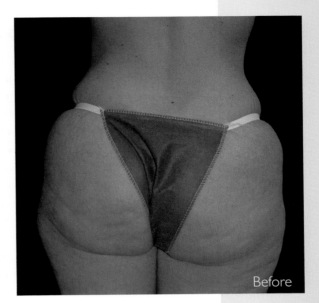

Before

Before

Age: 30

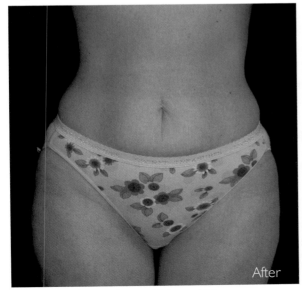
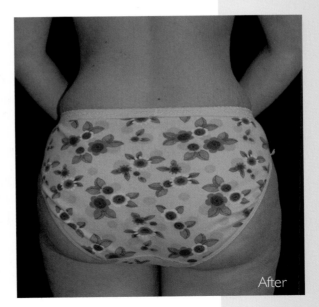

After

After

Procedure: liposuction to thighs and hips

> "The most important factor in recovery from liposuction is patience. Swelling and bruising are to be expected and can be severe. If often takes up to eight weeks for the majority of the swelling to dissipate. In other words you will usually look worse before you look better."
>
> —Steven Seidel, M.D.

Improvements in Liposuction Techniques

The suction tube used in liposuction is called a cannula, or liposuction rod. Cannulas resemble long, thin tubes (think of a drinking straw) and feature a blunt end with a hole through which fat is suctioned out of the body. The instruments are available in a number of sizes based on their length and diameter.

When liposuction was first introduced, surgeons used cannulas with large diameters that allowed for more fat to be removed in a shorter amount of time. Although they saved time, the large cannulas often produced undesirable results, including irregularities such as waviness or lumpiness. Over time, surgeons started using cannulas with smaller diameters, which allow for more precision in fat removal and body contouring. Using the smaller cannulas requires more time in the operating room, but generally results in a more pleasing, even contour. Whether your surgeon chooses a larger or smaller cannula may depend on the area being treated or the type of anesthesia or sedation used.

Depending on your surgeon's preference, the cannula will be attached to either a vacuum pump or a large syringe to create suction. Some surgeons may also connect the cannula to a motor that moves the cannula within the fat. Called power-assisted liposuction, this is used mainly to reduce the amount of physical effort required by the surgeon to perform the procedure.

After Your Liposuction Procedure

Following your liposuction procedure, you will most likely be placed in a compression garment that covers the treated areas. Depending on the areas treated, your compression garment may resemble bicycle shorts, a girdle, or leggings. This tight-fitting garment is designed to reduce swelling, relieve discomfort, and improve your final results. Some or all of your suctioned areas may also be covered with elastic tape or adhesive foam. Gauze dressings may be applied to the incision sites to absorb fluids as they drain.

Your stay in the recovery room will last approximately one to two hours. However, if you've had large-volume liposuction, you may require an overnight stay in a hospital or overnight facility. Once the anesthetic has worn off, and you're fully awake, you may go home. Under no circumstances will you be allowed to drive after surgery, so be sure you've arranged for a driver and at-home caregiver as detailed in your preoperative instructions.

Common Postsurgical Instructions

It is extremely important to follow any postsurgical instructions your surgeon gives you. The instructions you receive following liposuction will depend on several factors, including the areas treated, the volume of fat removed, and your surgeon's own experience and preferences. Here is a list of common postoperative instructions for liposuction.

- Wear your compression garment at all times for anywhere from one to six weeks. For your convenience, the garment has strategic cutouts to allow you to use the bathroom without removing it.

- You may shower within a few days after surgery. It's okay to remove the compression garment while you shower. (You may wash the garment when necessary.)

- Begin walking immediately. Be sure to walk every few hours while awake to avoid blood clots in the legs.

- Peel off any elastic tape or adhesive foam from the suctioned areas when instructed to do so, usually after a few days. It's easier to peel it off in the shower rather than "dry."

- Avoid vigorous exercise for at least two weeks.

- Because treated areas may feel numb, you may not realize that you are causing frostbite to your skin by leaving ice on too long.

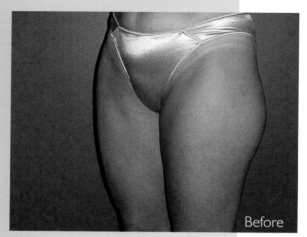

Age: 30

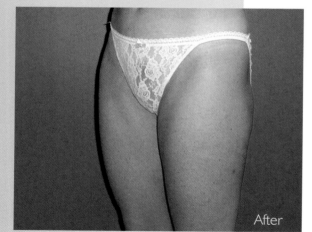

Procedure: Liposuction of thighs

- Change any gauze dressings on the incisions as instructed.

- Don't lift anything heavier than about five pounds until instructed otherwise.

- Continue taking any medications or supplements, such as iron pills, recommended by your surgeon.

In the Days and Weeks Ahead

Within the first few days after liposuction, you may have your first follow-up visit. During this visit, your surgeon will remove the compression garment and any dressings to examine the treated areas. After the examination, you'll put the garment back on and continue wearing it as instructed. Most likely, gauze dressings will no longer be necessary after a few days.

Any stitches will be removed at a subsequent follow-up visit approximately one week after your procedure. Upon examination, your surgeon will give you further instructions regarding the compression garment. At some point during your recovery, your surgeon may allow you to forego the garment in favor of tight-fitting spandex exercise shorts or pants.

As your recovery continues, your life will return to normal. You can generally return to office work within a week, but vigorous activities and aerobic exercise are not advised for at least two weeks. If you've had large-volume liposuction, your return to work, normal activities, and exercise may require more time.

Common Side Effects

Following liposuction, you may experience some common side effects associated with the procedure. If you've had liposuction performed on your hips, thighs, arms, or lower legs, it's important to realize that each side or limb will heal independently. You may experience certain side effects in only one of your arms or legs or only on one side. Likewise, the intensity of the symptoms may vary from side to side or from limb to limb.

- *Pain and discomfort:* The amount of pain felt in the treated areas following liposuction is highly individual but usually falls within the mild to moderate range. Pain medication prescribed by your doctor should alleviate any discomfort. If pain is severe or medication doesn't ease your pain, contact your doctor.

- *Lightheadedness and headaches:* A feeling of lightheadedness and pounding headaches may occur initially. These should subside within a few days.

- *Swelling:* Swelling in the treated areas is to be expected and usually peaks around three days after surgery. Don't be alarmed if swelling also occurs in hands, feet, or in some cases, genitalia. This is normal and will subside. You should see a vast decrease in swelling after one month, but it may take as much as six to nine months to disappear completely. Wearing the compression garment will help reduce swelling.

- *Bruising:* You can expect to have bruising in the treated areas. Bruising will decrease substantially within three to four weeks, but may take as long as six weeks to fade completely.

- *Altered sensation:* Any numbness or heightened sensitivity you experience in the treated areas will usually disappear within a few weeks.

- *Lumpiness:* During the recovery process, the suctioned areas may feel lumpy or irregular. This generally decreases over time. Massaging the treated areas may speed the process.

Risks and Potential Complications

In many cases, the risks and complications associated with liposuction may be attributed to a doctor's inexperience. Because of this, it is imperative to find a qualified, experienced, board-certified plastic surgeon to perform your procedure. However, even with the

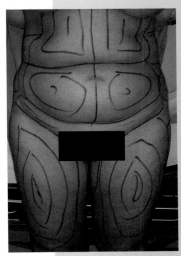

This woman is having liposuction of the abdomen, hips, sides, inner thighs, and inner knees.

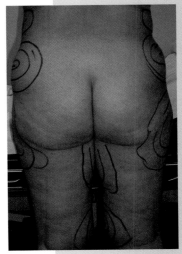

A plastic surgeon has applied markings that will serve as a guide for the areas undergoing liposuction.

Questions to Ask about Liposuction

- Which liposuction technique do you recommend for me and why?

- Where will the incisions be made?

- What size cannulas do you use and why?

- What is your reoperation rate?

- What are the most common reasons for reoperation?

- How much fat do you anticipate removing from me?

- Will I need a blood transfusion?

- How much experience do you have with this procedure?

- Is my skin tone adequate to get optimal results?

best plastic surgeon performing your procedure, complications may occur. With large-volume liposuction, complications are more likely.

- *Unevenness/skin irregularities*: Your final outcome may include unevenness or skin irregularities, such as waviness, wrinkling, or dimpling. Take heart that this potential problem is far less common these days thanks to the use of smaller cannulas during the procedure. However, if your skin had any of these conditions prior to surgery, you are more likely to experience them after your procedure.

- *Asymmetry*: Despite your surgeon's best efforts, your results may not be exactly alike on both sides. Some differences may be due to temporary swelling or lumpiness. If unacceptable differences remain after about six months, you may require a touch-up procedure to minimize the asymmetry.

- *Indentations/depressions*: When too much fat is removed from a specific area, it leaves an indentation or depression. This condition is difficult to correct and may require additional surgery to add fat back to the area.

- *Undercorrection*: To avoid indentations, surgeons prefer to be conservative with fat removal, which can result in undercorrection. A second surgery to remove additional fat may be recommended.

- *Deep venous thrombosis (DVT)/pulmonary embolism (PE)*: Failure to walk following surgery can lead to DVT (a blood clot in the deep veins of the thigh). A blood clot can travel through the body and lodge in the lungs, creating a very rare complication called pulmonary embolism. This potentially fatal complication can cause severe breathing problems.

- *Shock*: If the fluids lost during liposuction are not adequately replaced, it can lead to shock, which can be fatal in extremely rare cases. Shock is more commonly associated with large-volume liposuction, in which larger amounts of fluids are lost. Your surgeon may request that you donate your own blood prior to large-volume liposuction in case a transfusion is needed to reduce the risk of shock.

- *Fluid overload*: In rare instances, the tumescent fluid and other IV fluids given during liposuction can cause fluid overload. If your overall health is good, these fluids are absorbed by the body. But if you have a weak heart, fluid overload can lead to heart failure.

- *Nerve, tissue, or organ damage*: The cannulas used in liposuction can cause damage to nearby nerves, connective tissues, or organs.

- *Burns*: The heat generated by ultrasonic probes used in ultrasound-assisted liposuction can burn the skin if administered too long.

- *Lidocaine overdose*: Lidocaine, the local anesthetic, can be toxic if the dosage is excessive.

How Long Do Liposuction Results Last?

The removal of fat is permanent, as are the changes in your body contour. And unless you experience complications, suctioned areas will not require any specific ongoing follow-up care after you're fully healed. However, you must realize that liposuction doesn't give you free license to eat whatever you want or to be a couch potato. If you do put on pounds following the procedure, fat distribution can be unpredictable. The fat may or may not be distributed as proportionately as it was before your procedure. Participating in a regular exercise program and eating a proper diet are essential to maintaining your new and improved appearance.

CHAPTER EIGHT

Tummy Tuck

8

Tummy Tuck

*D*o you have a problem with a flabby abdomen? Are you frustrated that you still have loose skin and bulges in spite of all those sit-ups? Ideally, you would be able to achieve a trim and taut midsection by following a healthy diet and exercising regularly. Unfortunately, sometimes even the strictest diet and most vigorous workout routine can't deliver the look you want. And despite all your efforts, you may still have a bulging belly.

Fortunately, cosmetic plastic surgery has an answer to this common abdominal problem. It's called a tummy tuck, and it's one of the most sought-after body contouring procedures available. Each year, more than 150,000 people—at least 95 percent of them women—have the procedure and emerge with a flatter, more attractive abdomen. If you'd like to improve the appearance of your midsection, you may want to learn more about tummy tucks.

Basic Types of Tummy Tucks

To help you achieve a more svelte waistline, your surgeon can choose from several types of tummy tucks. The specific variation your surgeon chooses depends largely on the amount and location of excess loose skin and fat to be removed and the degree of weakness or separation of the muscles of the abdominal wall, called the rectus muscles.

Standard Tummy Tuck

The most commonly performed tummy tuck is called a standard tummy tuck. Like its name suggests, it is considered the standard technique for the procedure. All other types of tummy tucks are simply variations of the standard tummy tuck. This procedure is most appropriate when you have localized fat deposits, weakened rectus muscles, and excess skin on both the lower and upper abdomen. A standard tummy tuck removes excess skin and fat from below the belly button, tightens the rectus muscles, and pulls the remaining skin from the upper abdomen down to create tighter skin. With this procedure, your belly button will be surgically repositioned.

Extended Tummy Tuck

An extended tummy tuck may be recommended when saggy skin and bulges extend beyond the abdomen to the hips or back. The incision for an extended tummy tuck goes beyond that of a standard tummy tuck. With an extended tummy tuck, excess skin and fat are removed from each of the problem areas and skin is pulled down from above to create a smoother appearance. Tightening of the rectus muscles and navel repositioning are routinely performed with this variation of the procedure.

Mini Tummy Tuck

When a small amount of excess skin and fat is confined to the area below the belly button, a mini tummy tuck may be recommended. With this procedure, excess skin and fat are removed from below the navel, and weakened rectus muscles may also be tightened if necessary. With this procedure, your belly button isn't moved surgically, but it may end up in a slightly lower position on your abdomen.

Endoscopic Tummy Tuck

Designed primarily for thin women who have lax rectus muscles, the endoscopic tummy tuck tightens rectus muscles but

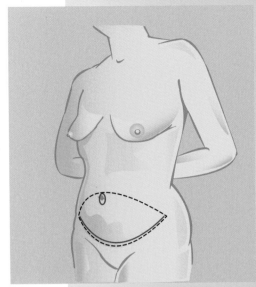

Incision for standard tummy tuck

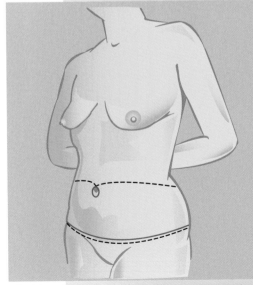

Incision placement for extended tummy tuck

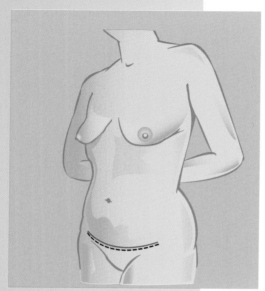

Incision for mini tummy tuck

doesn't remove excess skin or fat. This procedure is rarely performed in the United States. The reason it's seldom performed isn't due to any flaw in the procedure, but simply because American women generally don't fit this description. American women who have lax rectus muscles tend to also have loose skin and excess fat.

Are You a Candidate for a Tummy Tuck?

If you have a bulging belly, loose stomach skin, or lax abdominal muscles, you may be a candidate for a tummy tuck. A tummy tuck can be performed regardless of your age. Excellent results can be achieved whether you're twenty years old or in your golden years. More important than your age is your overall health and the shape of your body. The best candidates for this procedure have overall good health, have stabilized their weight, and are at or near their ideal weight but have localized fat deposits on the abdomen combined with loose skin and possibly lax abdominal muscles.

Only your surgeon can determine if you are indeed a candidate for a tummy tuck. To see if you can benefit from this procedure, your surgeon may have you bend over from the waist, tighten your abdominal muscles and then relax them. The amount of skin and fat that can be pinched in this position will help determine if a tummy tuck is the right procedure for you.

Good reasons candidates have for wanting a tummy tuck include the following.

- Multiple pregnancies: A tummy tuck can be particularly beneficial in reversing the effects of pregnancy on abdominal skin.
- Stretch marks: In addition to removing excess fat and skin, a tummy tuck may eliminate or significantly reduce stretch marks, especially if they are located on your lower abdomen.

- Weight fluctuations: Weight gain can stretch the skin to such a point that it loses its ability to contract. If this is the case, weight loss can leave you with unsightly, sagging skin that can't be improved with liposuction but can be treated with a tummy tuck.

- Aging and gravity: Aging and gravity can take their toll on abdominal skin, leaving it droopy and unattractive.

When a Tummy Tuck May Not Be for You

A tummy tuck can produce amazing results, but in some instances, it may not be right for you. For example, it may not achieve the results you want, or your surgeon may advise you to delay surgery for some time.

- If you have certain medical conditions: Health conditions that could prevent you from being a good candidate for a tummy tuck include heart disease, diabetes, or a history of blood clots. Having one of these medical conditions doesn't mean you will be denied a tummy tuck automatically. Your particular case will be evaluated by your surgeon, who may suggest additional testing before agreeing to take you on as a tummy-tuck patient.

- If you're a smoker: With any cosmetic surgery, smoking compromises skin circulation and healing and can lead to skin death at incision sites. Because the incisions associated with a tummy tuck are much larger than those associated with most other cosmetic procedures, the possibility of experiencing such complications is much higher for smokers.

- If you are obese: A tummy tuck is not a solution for obesity. Your doctor is likely to recommend diet and exercise or a surgical procedure, such as gastric bypass, as a means of weight loss. Following weight loss, a tummy tuck may be an option for you.

- If you have excess fat on your upper abdomen: If you carry a lot of fat on your upper abdomen as well as on your lower abdomen, your tummy-tuck results may not be optimal. Your doctor may suggest you lose weight prior to the procedure or may recommend liposuction of the upper abdomen in addition to a tummy tuck. Depending on your

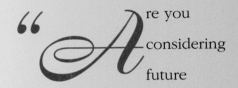

"Are you considering future pregnancies? If so, it's recommended that you postpone a tummy tuck until after you're finished having children."

—Thomas B. McNemar, M.D.

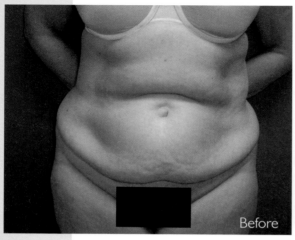

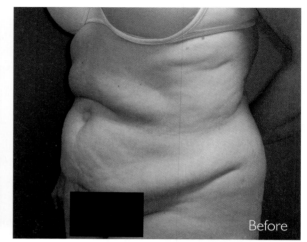

Before

Before

Age: 54. Height: 5' 5"
Weight: 178

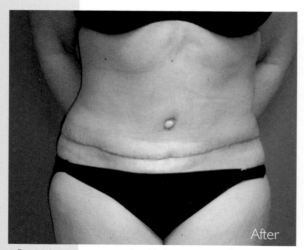

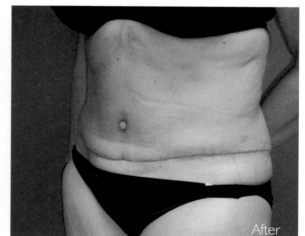

After

After

Procedure: tummy tuck with liposuction of abdomen
and flanks. Six weeks postoperative

surgeon, the two procedures may be done in the same operation or several months apart. In order to leave you with the tightest skin possible, your surgeon may suggest undergoing liposuction first, then having the tummy tuck at a later date.

- If you have intra-abdominal fat: A tummy tuck can't remove intra-abdominal fat, which is fat that is located throughout the intestines. Your surgeon can determine if you fall into this category and may suggest weight loss as an alternative.

- If you recently lost weight or intend to lose weight: Doctors recommend that your weight be stabilized for about six months prior to tummy-tuck surgery and that you maintain that weight following the procedure.

- If you plan to get pregnant: Your doctor will advise you to wait until after a pregnancy to have a tummy tuck. Pregnancy can cause skin and abdominal muscles that were tightened during a tummy tuck to stretch again and lose their contour, requiring additional tightening.

- If you have previous scars on the upper abdomen: Previous scars located above the area where skin and fat will be removed don't categorically disqualify you for a tummy tuck, but they could cause problems with healing. If there isn't enough skin circulation in the scarred area, it could lead to complications, such as skin death. Only your surgeon can determine if scars are problematic.

- If the idea of a long, permanent scar is unacceptable to you: Anyone considering a tummy tuck should be aware that the procedure leaves permanent scars. The scars are usually located just above the pubic bone on the lower abdomen and can extend from hip to hip or even beyond. In most cases, the scars can be hidden by underwear or a bathing suit. But, you may decide that lengthy scars are not an acceptable trade-off for a flatter stomach. In the end, only you can decide if living with the scar is worth the benefits of a tightened abdomen and more defined waist.

Your Tummy-Tuck Procedure

Standard Tummy Tuck

On average, a standard tummy-tuck procedure takes two to five hours. The operation involves several basic steps.

- Depending on your surgeon's preference, you may or may not be placed in compressive leg garments. These help promote blood flow throughout the legs and reduce the possibility of blood clots forming in the legs.

- Any liposuction being performed is done prior to making the tummy-tuck incisions.

- An incision is made around the navel as a way to release it from the surrounding tissue. A new opening is created in the skin for insertion of the belly button, which is stitched into a natural-looking position.

- A horizontal incision is made within or above the pubic area. This incision generally goes from hip bone to hip bone in either the shape of a smile or the letter W.

- The skin and underlying fat are pulled up and away from the body up to the rib cage, revealing the abdominal wall below.

- The connective tissues, or fascia, covering the rectus muscles are pulled together and tightened by stitching them together with permanent sutures or staples.

- The lifted abdominal skin is pulled and stretched down into its optimum position, and any excess skin and fat are trimmed away.

- Plastic drains are usually inserted prior to closing the incision to allow for postoperative draining.

- The incision is closed using either absorbable or nonabsorbable sutures below the skin. Surgical tape may be placed on the incision or additional external sutures may be used to help keep the incision closed.

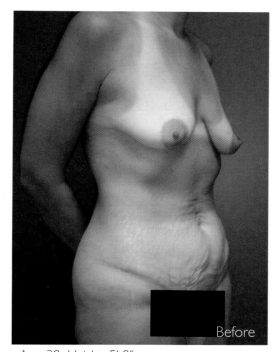

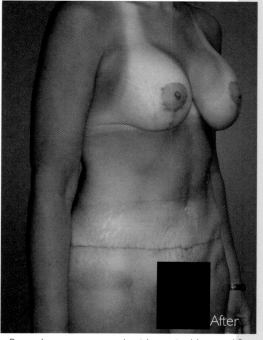

Age: 39. Height: 5' 9"
Weight: 164. Bra size: 36 B

Procedure: tummy tuck with vertical breast lift
with augmentation. Bra size: 36DD
Two months postoperative

Mini Tummy Tuck

A mini tummy-tuck procedure may take only one to two hours. The procedure is similar to the standard tummy tuck, except for the following.

- The horizontal incision is much shorter.

- Abdominal skin and fat are lifted away from the body only up to the navel.

- The connective tissues covering the rectus muscles may or may not be tightened, depending on individual needs.

- The navel is not repositioned.

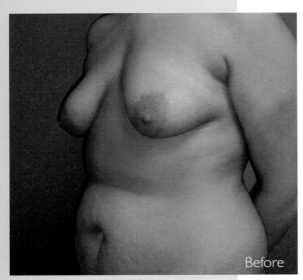

Age: 25. Height: 5' 6"
Weight: 143. Bra size: 36 B

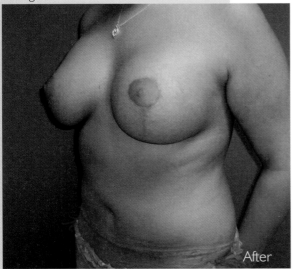

Procedure: tummy tuck with vertical breast lift with augmentation. Bra size: 36 D. Six weeks postoperative

Extended Tummy Tuck

An extended tummy tuck generally takes longer than a standard tummy tuck. It varies from the standard procedure in the following ways.

- The horizontal scar extends beyond the hip bones and as far around the body as the surgeon determines necessary. The incision may extend to include the hip areas and lower back, or it may encircle the entire body; however, the procedure then becomes a form of bodylift.

- The skin and underlying fat are lifted away from the hips and possibly from the back area as well.

- Excess skin and fat are also trimmed from the hips and possibly from the back area.

Endoscopic Tummy Tuck

An endoscopic tummy tuck is a much less invasive procedure than the standard tummy tuck. In this procedure, a small incision of only a few inches wide is made and an endoscope is inserted.

- The endoscope is a probe fitted with a fiber-optic camera that makes the vertical muscles of the abdominal wall visible through a small incision.

- The connective tissues covering the rectus muscles are tightened by stitching them together with permanent sutures or staples.

- In this procedure, no excess skin is removed, the navel isn't repositioned, and drains aren't necessary.

Your Tummy Tuck Incision

The incisions for a standard tummy-tuck procedure generally run from hip to hip between the pubic bone and the lower abdomen. These lengthy incisions leave lasting scars. Your surgeon will make every effort to keep the incisions within underwear or bathing-suit lines, but this isn't always possible. If there is a particular style of underwear or bathing suit you prefer to wear, talk to your surgeon about it before your surgery, or wear the garment to a preoperative visit to show your surgeon. It may be possible to make the incision in such a way that it will be hidden beneath the garment. If the navel is repositioned, a visible scar will surround it.

If you have an existing horizontal scar from a C-section (Cesarean section), your surgeon may be able to go through it for the tummy tuck, extending it as necessary. In some instances, it may be possible to eliminate an unsightly C-section scar that is red, raised, or uneven. By making the tummy-tuck incision below the existing scar, the scar can be removed completely along with the excess skin and fat.

Combining a Tummy Tuck with Other Procedures

A tummy tuck can be performed alone or it can be combined with other procedures. If you're hoping to make dramatic changes to your body contours, you may want to combine a tummy tuck with a thigh lift, buttock lift, or total body lift. You can also see a vastly improved silhouette by combining a tummy tuck with liposuction of the abdomen, hips, thighs, or buttocks.

However, there is some debate within the medical community about the safety of performing liposuction on the abdomen in conjunction with a tummy tuck, specifically regarding the amount and location of fat to be removed on the abdomen. It has been suggested that adding liposuction to the procedure may compromise blood flow to the skin and could lead to healing problems, including skin death. Some surgeons think the increased risks outweigh the benefits and recommend you wait several months after a tummy tuck to refine the contours of your tightened abdomen with liposuction. Other surgeons choose to perform limited amounts of liposuction on the abdomen in conjunction with a tummy tuck. Discuss these options with your surgeon.

> *I*f you're recovering from an abdominoplasty, you need to protect the abdominal wall from excess motion or strain in order to limit the amount of swelling and ultimately affect the outcome."
>
> —C. Andrew Salzberg, M.D.

In addition to performing a tummy tuck with other cosmetic procedures, it can also be combined with a hysterectomy, which is a medically necessary procedure. In this scenario, a gynecologic surgeon performs the hysterectomy, then the plastic surgeon steps in to tighten the abdomen with a tummy tuck. Most likely, the same incision will be used for both procedures, but it may need to be extended for the tummy tuck.

If you're hoping to have a tummy tuck immediately following childbirth, you should be aware that most surgeons discourage this practice. It is generally recommended that you wait at least six months following delivery before considering a tummy tuck.

After Tummy Tuck Surgery

Following your tummy-tuck procedure, you will probably be required to stay overnight in the surgical facility or hospital, but in some instances, you may be allowed to return home after a few hours in the recovery room. The length of your stay in the recovery room, surgical facility, or hospital depends on surgeon preference and the type of tummy tuck you have. For instance, if you have a mini tummy tuck, you're more likely to be allowed to return home on the day of surgery. Once you are home, it is recommended that you have a caregiver or responsible adult care for you for one to three days.

After your surgery, you may be outfitted with a number of surgical accessories, including compression hose, drainage tubes, a urinary catheter, gauze dressings, and Steri-Strips or surgical tape, and an abdominal binder. The abdominal binder is an elastic garment designed to reduce swelling, provide gentle pressure, and increase comfort level as you heal.

If a catheter is used, it will probably be for only the overnight stay in the surgical center. In an effort to avoid blood clots in your legs, your surgeon may choose to have you remain in the compression hose used during surgery. To prevent fluid collection under the skin, drainage tubes will be placed in the surgical area. At the end of each tube is a bulb, or reservoir, that collects fluids as they drain from the body. With a standard tummy tuck, you will usually have two drains. Steri-Strips or gauze dressings may be used on the incision sites.

You may also be sent home with a breathing device called an incentive spirometer. Following a tummy tuck, you may find that you don't want to breathe deeply because of pain and increased pressure in the abdominal area. The problem with this is that breathing shallowly for extended periods of time can put you at risk for pneumonia. The incentive spirometer helps prevent pneumonia by forcing you to breathe deeply.

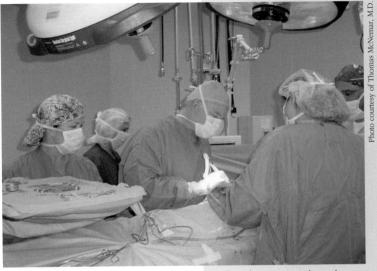

Photo courtesy of Thomas McNemar, M.D.

Tummy tuck surgery, underway here, usually takes two to three hours. This patient has received general anesthesia.

Common Postsurgical Instructions

To ensure a smooth recovery and to speed healing, your surgeon will provide you with detailed postoperative instructions. The specific instructions you receive depend on the type of tummy tuck performed as well as your surgeon's personal preferences and experience. To keep the healing process on track, it's imperative to follow the instructions meticulously. If there are any instructions you don't understand, ask your doctor. Here is a list of common postsurgical instructions for a tummy tuck.

- Wear your abdominal binder day and night for approximately two to six weeks or until instructed otherwise. You may remove the binder while showering and also to wash the garment. The binder should be snug but not constricting. If it feels too tight or causes pain, take it off. A binder that is too tight could interfere with skin circulation, possibly causing blistering or skin loss.

- Empty the bulbs on your drainage tubes as frequently as necessary. Every time you empty the bulbs, record the amount of

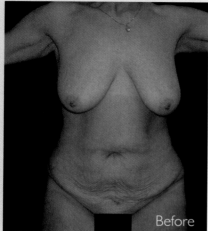

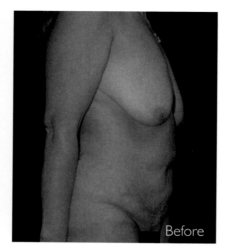

Age: 43. Height: 5'5"
Weight: 143

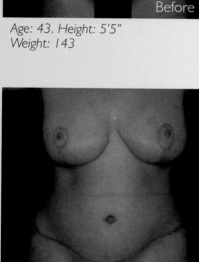

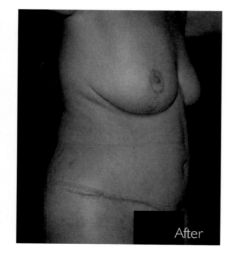

Procedure: tummy tuck with anchor
breast lift with augmentation
Eight weeks postoperative

fluid in each bulb so you can give this information to your doctor. The amount and color of the drainage will be taken into account as your doctor determines when the tubes can be removed.

- If you were sent home with compression hose and a pump machine, you will be required to wear the hose with the pump turned on at all times while at rest until instructed otherwise.

- Don't lie flat. Use a recliner at home with ample pillows to keep your head elevated and your knees bent. Likewise, in bed, keep your head and knees propped up with pillows.

- Standing up straight may be difficult for a week or two or even longer. Don't attempt to stretch or pull the abdomen straight during the first two to three weeks of healing.

- Once you return home, walking is mandatory to reduce the danger of blood clots in the legs. Get up and walk every few hours during the day. Because tightness in the abdomen makes it difficult to stand up straight at first, you may walk bent over. Increase the distance walked daily.

- Don't lift anything heavier than a glass of water for the first week.

- Don't strain or stoop down to pick up anything.

- You may shower within a day or two after surgery, but you should avoid soaking in a bathtub until the drainage tubes have been removed.

- If you have Steri-Strips or surgical tape on your incision, don't attempt to remove them. They will eventually fall off on their own. When showering, don't rub them vigorously with a washcloth or towel.

- If your doctor provides you with an incentive spirometer, use it at least ten times per hour during the day.

- Avoid vigorous exercise for approximately six weeks.

- Continue taking any medications, supplements, or over-the-counter remedies recommended by your surgeon. For instance, laxatives may be prescribed so you can avoid straining in the bathroom.

In the Days and Weeks Ahead

You will probably have several follow-up visits with your surgeon as you recover in the days and weeks following your surgery. Stitches from around the navel may be removed within the first week after surgery, but deeper sutures may not be removed for two to four weeks. Your drains will probably be removed within a week or two following your procedure. Your surgeon may allow you to stop wearing the binder after a few weeks or may require you to continue wearing it for several more weeks. Even if your doctor decides that you no longer need the binder, you may choose to continue wearing it if it makes you more comfortable.

Common Side Effects

During your recovery from a tummy tuck, you may experience certain side effects that are commonly associated with the procedure.

- *Pain*: The pain felt following a tummy tuck falls in the moderate to severe category and is sometimes compared to what you might experience following a C-section. However, a tummy tuck

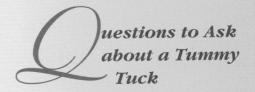

Questions to Ask about a Tummy Tuck

- Would I benefit more from liposuction or a tummy tuck?

- Which type of tummy tuck is right for me?

- How long will my scar be?

- Can my scars be hidden beneath underwear or a bathing suit?

- Will you be able to remove my stretch marks?

- What is your reoperation rate?

- What are the most common reasons for reoperation?

- What if I gain weight after the procedure?

- What if I get pregnant after the procedure?

- Will I have to stay overnight following the procedure?

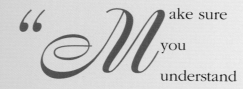

"*M*ake sure you understand the tummy tuck's scar placement. You are trading a flatter stomach for the long scar."

—Thomas B. McNemar, M.D.

may actually prove to be less painful than a C-section because the latter procedure is a more invasive operation, involving the abdominal cavity and uterus as well. The tightening of the muscles of the abdominal wall is generally considered the most painful aspect of a tummy tuck.

- *Swelling*: In general, swelling will peak about three days after surgery. You can expect most of the swelling to dissipate within a month, but it may take several months for it to disappear completely. Don't be alarmed if swelling involves your hands and feet as well as your abdomen.

- *Tightness*: If your tummy tuck involves tightening of the muscles of the abdominal wall, you can expect to feel tightness in this area for a month or longer.

- *Discoloration*: Any bruising or discoloration of the surgical area will be temporary.

- *Numbness*: You may experience a feeling of numbness in the abdominal skin for several months or even longer. It may take as long as two years for sensation in your abdomen to be fully restored.

- *Tingling, burning, and shooting pains*: If you feel tingling, burning, or shooting pains, don't be alarmed. This feeling simply indicates regeneration of the small sensory nerves in the surgical area and will disappear with time.

- *Feeling of fullness*: When you eat, you may find that you feel full sooner than normal.

Risks and Potential Complications

Although the great majority of tummy-tuck patients express satisfaction with their results, there are risks associated with the procedure. Complications are less likely with mini–tummy tucks and endoscopic tummy tucks because they are less invasive and involve much smaller incisions.

- *"Dog ears"*: In addition to the possible scarring complications associated with any surgery, a tummy-tuck scar may also form what's called a dog ear. This occurs when a surgeon closes the horizontal incision and a small flap of bulging tissue is formed at the ends of the incision. The dog ear may flatten or disappear with time. If it doesn't, it may require an additional procedure performed under local anesthesia.

- *Surface lumps/irregularities*: The skin contours of the abdomen may be slightly uneven or asymmetrical, and slight depressions or wrinkling can occur. Most of these problems will improve dramatically on their own.

- *Deep venous thrombosis (DVT)/pulmonary embolism (PE)*: Failure to walk following surgery can lead to DVT (a blood clot in the deep veins of the thigh). A blood clot can travel through the body and lodge in the lungs, creating a very rare complication called pulmonary embolism. This potentially fatal complication can cause severe breathing problems.

- *Belly-button problems*: If the navel is repositioned, it may be slightly off center, or it might protrude or be unusually retracted following surgery.

- *Fat necrosis*: In rare cases, skin that is pulled too tight or an infection can cause underlying fat to die. When this occurs, additional healing time is necessary, but it doesn't usually affect the ultimate outcome of the procedure. Smokers are more at risk for fat necrosis. Signs of fat necrosis include hard nodules or firmness under the skin. Treatment may include drainage and, in severe cases, additional surgery.

Follow-Up Care

After you're fully healed, your streamlined abdomen won't require any specific follow-up care. You'll probably begin to see what your new

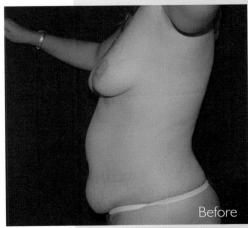

Age: 34. Height 5'3"
Weight: 139 pounds

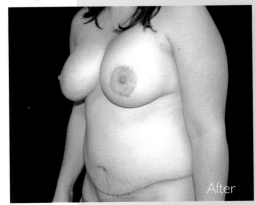

Procedure: tummy tuck and breast lift with augmentation. Eight weeks postoperative

contours will look like after swelling subsides within a few months. After about a year, when your scars have faded, you'll see the final results.

How Long Does a Tummy Tuck Last?

A tummy tuck is considered a permanent procedure. Excess skin and fat are permanently removed, and the tightening of the abdominal wall is also a lasting solution. However, if you gain weight or go through a pregnancy following the procedure, your skin and abdominal wall may stretch and become loose again, requiring additional tightening. Although pregnancy can reverse the effects of a tummy tuck, the procedure has no effect on your ability to become pregnant in the future and doesn't impact future pregnancies in any way. The good news is that if you maintain your weight, you should continue enjoying the results of your tummy tuck for years to come.

In Closing

We hope you have found the information in this book helpful in making an informed decision regarding breast augmentation and body contouring surgery. Although this book contains the most up-to-date information available, it's important to remember that it is only a starting point in your research. We encourage you to learn more by consulting other sources, such as those listed in the Resources section.

Most importantly, this book should not be considered a substitute for a consultation with a qualified plastic surgeon. If you're considering one of the surgical procedures covered in this book, we encourage you to make an appointment with a board-certified plastic surgeon. With the information in this book, you should be better equipped to ask the right questions during your consultation, to weigh the risks and rewards of surgery, and ultimately, to make the best choices regarding body-contouring surgery.

Accreditation Association for Ambulatory Health Care

3201 Old Glenview Road, Suite 300
Wilmette, IL 60091
Phone: 847-853-6060
www.aaahc.org

Formed in 1979, the Accreditation Association for Ambulatory Health Care (AAAHC), also known as the Accreditation Association, develops standards to advance patient safety, quality, and value through peer-based accreditation processes, education, and research. The peer-based program currently accredits more than 2,300 ambulatory-health-care organizations. Accreditation is on a voluntary basis, and organizations are evaluated based on nationally recognized standards developed by the AAAHC. The AAAHC's Web site allows you to search for accredited organizations and explains what accreditation means to you as a patient.

American Academy of Cosmetic Surgery

Cosmetic Surgery Information Service
737 North Michigan Avenue, Suite 2100
Chicago, IL 60611-5405
Phone: 312-981-6760
www.cosmeticsurgery.org

Founded in 1985, the American Academy of Cosmetic Surgery (AACS) is a professional medical society whose members include plastic surgeons, facial plastic surgeons, ocular plastic surgeons, dermatologic surgeons, head and neck surgeons, and general surgeons, among others. The AACS is the nation's largest organization representing cosmetic surgeons. The AACS is dedicated to patient safety and physician education in cosmetic surgery and offers ongoing postgraduate education specifically in cosmetic surgery. The Academy's Web site provides information on surgical procedures and the risks involved, explains how to choose a cosmetic surgeon, and offers a physician-finder service.

American Association for the Accreditation of Ambulatory Surgery Facilities, Inc.

5101 Washington Street, Suite 2F
Gurnee, IL 60031
Phone: 888-545-5222
www.aaaasf.org

Established in 1980, the American Association for the Accreditation of Ambulatory Surgery Facilities, Inc. (AAAASF) has developed an accrediting program to help provide patients with the assurance of safety and quality for their outpatient-surgery experience. To earn accreditation, surgery facilities must meet stringent national standards for equipment, operating-room safety, personnel, and surgeon credentials. The organization has developed a means of measuring medical and surgical competence as well as ethical conduct. The not-for-profit AAAASF has accredited more than one thousand outpatient surgical facilities. The AAAASF Web site allows you to search for accredited surgical facilities and explains the safety and quality standards that must be met.

American Board of Anesthesiology

4101 Lake Boone Trail, Suite 510
Raleigh, NC 27607
Phone: 919-881-2570
www.abanes.org

Formed in 1937, the American Board of Anesthesiology (ABA) examines and certifies physicians who complete an accredited program of anesthesiology training in the United States and voluntarily apply to the board for certification or maintenance of certification. Its mission is to maintain the highest standards in the practice of anesthesiology and to serve the public, medical profession, and health-care facilities and organizations. The organization fosters educational facilities and training in anesthesiology. A directory on the ABA Web site allows you to search for ABA diplomates and candidates.

American Board of Medical Specialties

1007 Church Street, Suite 404
Evanston, IL 60201-5913
Phone: 847-491-909
www.abms.org

Established in 1933, the American Board of Medical Specialties (ABMS) is a not-for-profit organization consisting of twenty-four approved medical specialty boards. It is the nation's preeminent entity overseeing physician certification. Board certification is intended to provide patients with assurance that a physician has completed an approved residency training program, has passed comprehensive examinations, and has met other board requirements. The ABMS Web site explains how specialists are trained and certified, and a search feature allows patients to find certified surgeons.

American Board of Plastic Surgery

Seven Penn Center, Suite 400
1635 Market Street
Philadelphia, PA 19103-2204
Phone: 215-587-9322
www.abplsurg.org

Initially organized in 1937, the American Board of Plastic Surgery (ABPS) is one of the twenty-four specialty boards recognized by the American Board of Medical Specialties. Created to promote safe and ethical plastic surgery, it offers certification only to physicians who specialize in plastic surgery. Certification requirements can be found on the organization's Web site.

American Society for Aesthetic Plastic Surgery

11081 Winners Circle
Los Alamitos, CA 90720
Phone: 888-ASAPS-11
or 888-272-7711 (physician referrals)
www.surgery.org/public/index.php

Founded in 1967, the American Society for Aesthetic Plastic Surgery (ASAPS) is the leading organization of board-certified plastic surgeons specializing in cosmetic plastic surgery. The ASAPS focuses its efforts on continuing education for qualified cosmetic plastic surgeons, public information, patient advocacy, and research. On the ASAPS Web site, the public can read the latest news regarding cosmetic surgery, locate a surgeon, view before-and-after photos, learn about procedures, and find the average costs for various procedures. The site also offers an "Ask the Surgeon" feature where the public can anonymously post questions to be answered by a board-certified cosmetic plastic surgeon.

American Society of Anesthesiologists

520 North Northwest Highway
Park Ridge, IL 60068-2573
Phone: 847-825-5586
www.asahq.org

Established in 1905, the American Society of Anesthesiologists (ASA) is an educational, research, and scientific association with more than thirty-eight thousand physician members. The ASA's goals include maintaining standards of the medical practice of anesthesiology and improving patient care. On the Web site, you'll find a patient-education section with useful and important information about the medical care you receive before, during, and after surgical procedures.

American Society of Plastic Surgeons

444 East Algonquin Road
Arlington Heights, IL 60005
Phone: 847-228-9900; 888-4-PLASTIC or 888-475-27842 (physician referrals)
www.plasticsurgery.org

Established in 1931, the American Society of Plastic Surgeons (ASPS) is the largest plastic-surgery specialty organization in the world. Composed of board-certified plastic surgeons who perform reconstructive and cosmetic surgery, the ASPS advocates for patient safety and encourages high standards of ethics, practice, and research. On the Web site, you can learn about various procedures, read patient testimonials. and view before-and-after photos. The *Plastic Surgery Today* patient newsletter and "Ask a Plastic Surgeon" chat feature are also available on the site.

Breastimplantsafety.org

(See also American Society of Plastic Surgeons and American Society for Aesthetic Plastic

Surgery)
www.breastimplantsafety.org

This authoritative resource on breast-implant safety comes from a collaboration of the American Society of Plastic Surgeons and the American Society for Aesthetic Plastic Surgery. This Web site offers information on the safety and risks associated with both saline and silicone implants and provides updates on clinical trials and the U.S. Food and Drug Administration's policies regarding implants. Additional patient information includes a list of questions to ask your surgeon about breast augmentation and links to the latest studies and articles on breast implants.

eMedicine, Inc.

Morgan Place, Suite 402
8420 West Dodge Road
Omaha, NE 68102
Phone: 402-341-3222
www.emedicine.com; www.emedicinehealth.com (for consumers)

Although designed for health professionals, the eMedicine Web site offers free access to hundreds of professional medical articles written by physicians. A portion of the Web site is dedicated solely to consumers and includes more than 6,500 pages of patient-education material. Within these pages, you can find detailed descriptions of hundreds of surgical procedures, including liposuction.

Healthfinder

P.O. Box 1133
Washington, DC 20013-1133
www.healthfinder.gov

Developed in 1997 by the U.S. Department of Health and Human Services together with other federal agencies, Healthfinder is a key resource for finding consumer health information. Healthfinder provides links to more than 1,500 health-related organizations. Topic searches will bring up news, feature articles, Web links, and related organizations.

Inamed Aesthetics

5540 Ekwill Street
Santa Barbara, CA 93111
Phone: 805-683-6761
www.inamed.com

One of the nation's leading manufacturers of breast implants for more than twenty-five years, Inamed Aesthetics (formerly known as McGhan Medical) offers details on breast-implant warranties and financial assistance in addition to in-depth patient information on its Web site. Comprehensive booklets on breast augmentation surgery and saline-filled implants are available for download and include statistics on patient satisfaction. The Web site also includes before-and-after photos, a physician-search feature, frequently asked questions, and updates on breast-implant issues.

Institute of Medicine

505 Fifth Street NW
Washington DC 20001
Phone: 202-334-2352
www.iom.edu

Chartered in 1970, the nonprofit Institute of
Medicine (IOM) serves as an adviser to the nation
in an effort to improve health. Working
independently of any government agency, the
organization provides unbiased, evidence-based,
and authoritative information and advice to policy
makers, professionals, and consumers. The
institute's Web site offers hundreds of reports,
studies, and analyses on various health issues,
including the safety of silicone breast implants.

Liposuction.com

1001 Avenida Pico, Suite C402
San Clemente, CA 92673
Phone: 949-369-7555
www.liposuction.com

This consumer-oriented Web site offers a history
of liposuction, an overview of the techniques
available, a discussion on safety and
complications, information on postoperative care,
average costs for the procedure, and more. The
site features numerous before-and-after photos of
liposuction from various areas of the body,
including the abdomen, hips, thighs, buttocks,
arms, and back. A surgeon directory allows you
to search for a qualified physician in your area.

Mentor Corporation

201 Mentor Drive
Santa Barbara, CA 93111
Phone: 800-525-0245; 800-636-8678
(for patient questions about aesthetics products)
www.mentor4me.com

Mentor Corporation is one of the leading
manufacturers of breast implants. Its
consumer-oriented site is a complete resource
center for women considering breast
augmentation. The site includes detailed
information on breast augmentation options, what
to expect, before-and-after photos, patient
testimonials, frequently asked questions, risks and
complications, clinical studies, and more.
Consumers can download a copy of their
informative brochure, *Saline-Filled Breast Implant
Surgery: Making an Informed Decision.*

National Women's Health Information Center

U.S. Department of Health and Human
Services/Office on Women's Health
8270 Willow Oaks Corporate Drive
Fairfax, VA 22031
Phone: 800-994-9662

Established in 1991, the National Women's Health
Information Center (NWHIC) offers free
women's-health information on more than eight
hundred topics. On the Web site, you can find
women's-health statistics, daily news, and articles
from thousands of health publications. A "Body
Image" section of the Web site provides a guide

to cosmetic-surgery procedures and their risks, as well as dozens of related articles.

National Women's Health Resource Center, Inc.

157 Broad Street, Suite 315
Red Bank, NJ 07701
Phone: 877-986-9472 (toll-free)
www.healthywomen.org

Since 1988, the National Women's Health Resource Center, Inc. (NWHRC) has been providing women with the information needed to educate themselves about important health topics. The nonprofit organization is a clearinghouse for reliable, unbiased women's-health information developed in collaboration with top health-care experts and organizations. Topics covered include liposuction and preparing for surgery.

U.S. Food and Drug Administration

5600 Fishers Lane
Rockville, MD 20857
Phone: 888-INFO-FDA or 888-463-6332
www.fda.gov/cdrh/breastimplants;
www.fda.gov/cdrh/liposuction

The U.S. Food and Drug Administration (FDA) is the agency that regulates cosmetic procedures, medications, breast implants, and the sale of medical devices, such as the cannulas and ultrasonic probes used for liposuction. The agency publishes the *FDA Breast Implant Consumer Handbook*, which is available for download on its Web site and includes detailed information about the various breast implants

available and what to expect from the surgical procedure. Consumers can also download brochures on breast-implant complications as well as the latest breast-implant studies. The Web site also provides an overview of liposuction, including a glossary of terms, risks, and complications, what to expect, who can perform liposuction, and how to report problems.

U.S. National Library of Medicine

8600 Rockville Pike
Bethesda, MD 20894
Phone: 888-FIND-NLM or 888-346-3656;
301-594-5983
www.nlm.nih.gov/medlineplus

Designed primarily for health professionals and scientists, the National Library of Medicine Web site, called MedlinePlus, is a gold mine of authoritative health information drawn from the National Library of Medicine, the National Institutes of Health, and other government agencies and health-related organizations. The site offers up-to-date health news, an illustrated medical encyclopedia, a medical dictionary, and interactive patient tutorials. Users can view articles on health-related topics from more than 3,500 medical journals and can search through more than 650 topics, including cosmetic surgery.

Glossary

abdominoplasty: the medical term for a tummy tuck

adrenaline: see *epinephrine*

anatomical implant (also called a teardrop, contoured, or shaped implant): a breast implant that is fuller on the bottom than on the top as opposed to being round (See also *breast implant.)*

anesthesia: any one of a number of methods used to induce relaxation and either drowsiness or a deep sleep in a patient during surgery to eliminate pain

areola: the shaded area surrounding the nipple

aspiration: a technique used to remove a hematoma or seroma by injecting a thin needlelike instrument

asymmetry: a condition in which there are differences between two sides, for instance, when two breasts differ in size, shape, or nipple position, or when the amount of fat in two thighs is unequal

autoimmune diseases: see *connective-tissue diseases*

belt lipectomy: a surgical procedure in which an incision is made around the body like a belt to remove excess skin and fat from the abdomen, hips, and back

body contouring: any cosmetic-surgery procedure that reshapes the body

breast augmentation: a surgical procedure that increases the size of the breasts by inserting an implant (See also *breast implant.)*

breast implant: a sac made of a rubberlike *silicone* shell that is filled with saline or silicone gel (See also *high-profile breast implant.)*

breast lift: a surgical procedure that lifts and reshapes saggy breasts

breast projection: the distance the breast tissue that projects forward from the chest

cannula: a long strawlike instrument used to suction fat during liposuction

capsular contracture: a complication following breast augmentation in which the scar tissue that normally forms in the capsule around the implant begins to contract and squeeze the implant

capsule: lining created by the body around a breast implant

capsule calcification: a condition in which calcium deposits develop in the capsule around the breast implant and may be mistaken for possible cancer on mammograms (See also *mammogram.)*

cc (cubic centimeter): a measure of volume used for filling breast implants

cellulite: puckered or dimpled skin usually appearing on the hips, thighs, or buttocks

collagen: a fibrous protein found in the connective tissues that supports the skin

connective tissue: tissue that supports and binds together other tissues, such as tendons, muscles, ligaments, bones, and cartilage

connective-tissue diseases (also called autoimmune diseases): diseases such as lupus, rheumatoid arthritis, rheumatic fever, fibromyalgia, and chronic fatigue syndrome, in which the body's own defense system attacks the connective tissues, creating inflammation or degenerative changes in those tissues

contoured implant: see *anatomical implant*

deep venous thrombosis (DVT): the formation of a blood clot within a deep vein, usually in the thigh

diastasis: the abnormal separation of the vertical muscles of the abdominal wall

dog ear: a complication in which tissue bulges at the end of a scar

Eklund technique: a series of additional X-rays taken during a *mammogram* in which the breast implant is pushed back and the breast tissue is pulled forward in an effort to improve detection of breast cancer

elastin: a protein that gives the skin its elasticity

elastomer: the rubberlike substance that is used to make breast-implant shells

electrocardiogram (EKG or ECG): a procedure used for diagnosing abnormal heartbeats

endoscope: a surgical probe equipped with a fiber-optic camera

epinephrine: also called *adrenaline*, this hormone is used in *tumescent liposuction* to constrict blood vessels, to prolong the effects of local anesthetics, and to reduce bleeding

estrogen: a hormone that promotes the development of the female breasts, among other functions

external ultrasound-assisted liposuction: a *liposuction* technique in which high-frequency sound waves are transmitted through the skin of the area to be treated

fascia: connective tissues that cover or bind together structures of the body, such as the muscles of the abdominal wall, the *rectus muscles*

flanks: the fleshy part of the body between the ribs and the hip

hematoma: a collection of blood within the tissue of the body

high-profile breast implant: a breast implant with a narrower diameter, designed to create greater projection and often used for small or petite women

incentive spirometer: a device used to encourage patients to breathe deeply following a surgical procedure as a way to prevent pneumonia

inframammary fold: the crease or fold beneath the breast

inframammary technique: a surgical technique in which a surgeon makes the incision for a breast augmentation procedure on or near the fold of the underside of the breast

intra-abdominal fat: fat that is interspersed throughout the abdominal organs

keloid: a thick, raised, uneven scar caused by excessive tissue growth at the site of a surgical incision or wound

lidocaine: a crystalline compound used in *tumescent liposuction* as a local anesthetic

liposuction: the surgical removal of localized fat deposits in the body by using suction through a small cannula

mammogram: a series of X-ray views used to detect cancer in the breasts (See also *Eklund technique.*)

mastopexy: the medical term for a *breast lift*

menopause: the cessation of menstruation, usually occurring between the ages of forty-five and fifty-five

metabolic rate: the pace at which your body creates and uses energy for vital functions, such as absorbing and processing nutrients, circulating blood, breathing, eliminating waste, and regulating body temperature

milk ducts: the tubular passages that carry milk produced in the *milk glands* to the nipples

milk glands: where milk is produced in the breasts

monitored anesthesia care (MAC): a technique in which an anesthesiologist sedates a patient while continuously monitoring his or her vital signs

necrosis: tissue death usually due to a loss of circulation

nipple/areola complex: the nipple and surrounding shaded area

pectoral muscle: the muscle located between the breasts and the ribs

periareolar technique: a surgical technique in which a surgeon makes the incision for a breast augmentation procedure along the outer edge of the areola

progesterone: a hormone that promotes the development of the female breasts, among other sexual-reproductive functions

ptosis: the medical term for sagging breasts

reconstructive surgery: surgery that is performed to restore function or normal appearance **the** muscles of the abdominal wall

rippling: see *wrinkling*

rupture: a complication in which a breast implant is punctured and may subsequently leak or deflate

saddlebags: disproportionate fat deposits located on the outer thighs

sedation: a method in which sedatives are administered to the patient to induce relaxation, drowsiness, or unconsciousness as a way to eliminate pain during a surgical procedure

seroma: a collection of clear fluid within the body

shaped implant: see *anatomical implant*

silicone: a rubberlike substance used to make the *breast-implant* sacs that are subsequently filled with *sterile saline* or *silicone gel*

silicone gel: a gelatinous substance made of *silicone* that is sometimes used to fill *breast implants*

sloshing: the sound of body fluids moving within the *capsule* created for a *breast implant*

sterile saline: a saltwater solution, similar to what is found in the human body, that is used to fill *breast implants*

Steri-Strips: a type of surgical tape that can be used in lieu of sutures to keep incisions closed

subcutaneous fat: the thick, deep layer of fat that responds best to *liposuction*

subglandular: the placement of a *breast implant* beneath the breast tissue but above the pectoral muscle

submuscular: the placement of a *breast implant* beneath the pectoral muscle

superficial fat: the thin layer of fat found directly beneath the skin that contributes to *cellulite*

synmastia: a complication following breast augmentation in which the skin detaches from the breastbone and the two breasts form the appearance of a single breast

teardrop implant: see *anatomical implant*

Toxic shock syndrome (TSS): an acute and sometimes fatal disease resulting from a bacterial infection, its symptoms include fever, nausea, and diarrhea

transaxillary technique: a surgical technique in which the incision for a breast augmentation procedure is made in the armpit area.

transumbilical technique: an *endoscopic* surgical technique in which a surgeon makes the incision for a breast augmentation procedure in the belly button

tuberous breasts: a condition in which the breasts have a long, narrow mound of breast tissue protruding from the chest wall

tumescent: a technique used in *liposuction* in which large amounts of fluids are injected into the area to be treated

tummy tuck: a surgical procedure in which excess skin and fat are permanently removed from the abdomen and muscles of the abdominal wall are tightened

ultrasonic liposuction: a liposuction technique that uses high-frequency sound waves

ultrasound: high-frequency sound waves

Wise pattern: a technique used for a breast lift in which incisions are made in the shape of an anchor or inverted T

wrinkling: a complication following breast augmentation in which waves of saline within the implant are visible through the skin, creating a wrinkling or *rippling* effect

Index

About the Authors

Thomas McNemar, M.D., is a plastic surgeon in private practice with offices in Tracy and San Ramon, California. He attended the Medical College of Ohio where he made the decision to pursue a surgical career. After completing a general surgery residency at the Cleveland Clinic, he continued his surgical education at Akron City Hospital as a plastic-surgery fellow. He rounded out his formal education at the Bunke Clinic in San Francisco, California, as an attending fellow specializing in hand and microvascular surgery.

Dr. McNemar is married and the father of two children. He and his family enjoy the outdoor leisure activities and fine-art opportunities the Bay area has to offer. He enjoys skiing, bicycling, and the culinary arts.

Dr. McNemar may be reached through his Web site: **www.drmcnemar.com**.

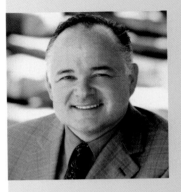

"Every patient is beautiful and unique. I believe that cosmetic surgery can renew and accentuate one's outer beauty, while enhancing inner beauty and a higher sense of self confidence."

—Thomas McNemar, M.D.

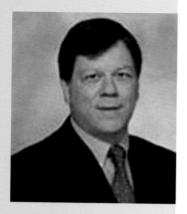

*"Cosmetic surgery has given joy
and meaning to my life. I'm
thankful for the ability to shape the
lives of so many people, and as I
educate patients each day, I,
myself, gain knowledge and
enlightenment."*
— C. Andrew Salzberg, M.D.

C. **Andrew Salzberg, M.D.,** specializes in cosmetic surgery and breast surgery was a partner in the New York Group for Plastic Surgery, LLP, in Westchester County, New York. He is also the chief of plastic surgery at Community Hospital at Dobbs Ferry and is an associate professor at Westchester Medical Center in New York.

Dr. Salzberg has been named one of the "Top Doctors for Women from Coast to Coast" by *America's Top Doctors*, a consumer guide published by *Ladies' Home Journal.* He was bestowed the honor of being named one of the top doctors in the New York Metro Area in 2002 to 2005.

Dr. Salzberg has been board-certified in plastic and reconstructive surgery since 1989. He has been an associate professor of plastic surgery and otolaryngology at New York Medical College since 1987. He served as chief of plastic and reconstructive surgery at the Castle Point VA Medical Center in New York from 1987 to 1997 and is a past president of the National Pressure Ulcer Advisory Panel.

Dr. Salzberg attended Montclair Academy in N.J. and Ithaca College in New York. He graduated from the University of Florida School of Medicine in 1981. He completed his residency in general surgery at Beth Israel Hospital and his plastic surgery residency at Mount Sinai Medical Center in New York. He has presented papers regarding plastic surgery internationally, and his research activities include breast reconstruction and he has recently pioneered an immediate one stage breast technique.

Dr. Salzberg may be reached through his Web site: **www.nygplasticsurgery.com**.

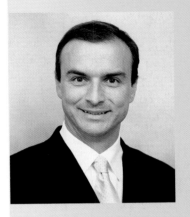

Steven P. Seidel, M.D., a plastic surgeon in private practice in Cullman, Alabama, is the director of Seidel Plastic Surgery, a freestanding cosmetic-surgery clinic, which he established in 1996. He also serves as chief of staff at Cullman Regional Medical Center.

Dr. Seidel graduated Phi Beta Kappa from the University of Wisconsin, Madison, with degrees in biochemistry and German literature. He completed a residency in general surgery at the University of Michigan and a plastic-surgery fellowship at the University of Alabama, Birmingham. Dr. Seidel holds board certification in general surgery as well as plastic surgery.

Dr. Seidel specializes in all major areas of cosmetic surgery, with an emphasis on breast augmentation, body contouring, and endoscopic surgery. He is the author of numerous published book chapters and scientific articles. He lives with his wife, Bethany, and three children in the Cullman area.

Dr. Seidel may be reached through his Web site: **seidelplasticsurgery.com** or by email: **sseidel@prn-inc.net.**

"My job is fascinating, in part, because every patient is different. Excellence in cosmetic surgery requires attention to detail and knowing your patients. Patients sense and appreciate that level of dedication and personal interest in them."

— Steven P. Seidel, M.D.

Consumer Health Titles

Visit our online catalog at www.AddicusBooks.com

After Mastectomy	$14.95
Body Contouring Surgery after Weight Loss	$24.95
Cancers of the Mouth and Throat	$14.95
Cataracts: A Patient's Guide to Treatment	$14.95
Colon & Rectal Cancer	$14.95
Coping with Psoriasis	$14.95
Coronary Heart Disease	$15.95
Countdown to Baby	$14.95
Exercising Through Your Pregnancy	$17.95
The Fertility Handbook	$14.95
The Macular Degeneration Source Book	$14.95
LASIK—A Guide to Laser Vision Correction	$14.95
Living with P.C.O.S.—Polycystic Ovarian Syndrome	$14.95
Lung Cancer—A Guide to Treatment & Diagnosis	$14.95
The Macular Degeneration Source Book	$14.95
The Non-Surgical Facelift Book	$19.95
Overcoming Metabolic Syndrome	$14.95
Overcoming Postpartum Depression and Anxiety	$14.95
A Patient's Guide to Dental Implants	$14.95
Prescription Drug Addiction—The Hidden Epidemic	$15.95
Prostate Cancer—A Patient's Guide to Treatment	$14.95
A Simple Guide to Thyroid Disorders	$14.95
Straight Talk About Breast Cancer	$14.95
The Stroke Recovery Book	$14.95
The Surgery Handbook	$14.95
Understanding Lumpectomy	$14.95
Understanding Parkinson's Disease	$14.95
Understanding Your Living Will	$12.95
Your Complete Guide to Breast Augmentation	$21.95
Your Complete Guide to Breast Reduction	$21.95
Your Complete Guide to Facial Cosmetic Surgery	$19.95
Your Complete Guide to Face Lifts	$21.95
Your Complete Guide to Nose Reshaping	$21.95